Tamilee Webb's
STEP UP
FITNESS
WORKOUT

Tamilee Webb's
STEP UP
FITNESS

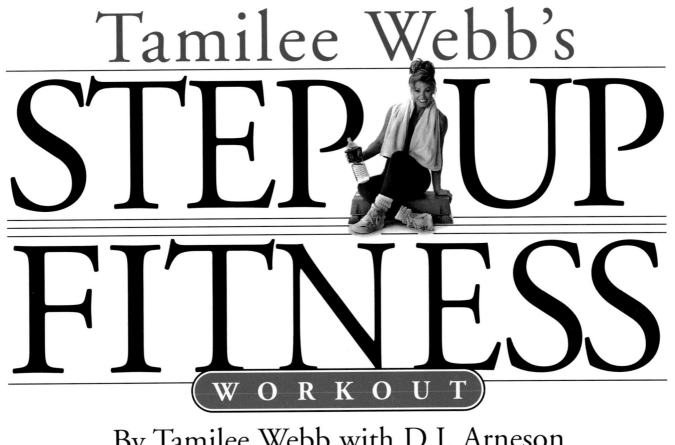

WORKOUT

By Tamilee Webb with D.J. Arneson

Photographs by Ellen Wallop

WORKMAN PUBLISHING, NEW YORK

Library of Congress
Cataloging-in-Publication Data

Webb, Tamilee
(Step Up Fitness Workout)
Tamilee Webb's Step Up Fitness Workout /
Tamilee Webb with D.J. Arneson;
photographs by Ellen Wallop.
p.cm
ISBN 1-56305-491-4
1. Step aerobics. I. Arneson, D.J. II. Wallop, Ellen. III. Title: Step up fitness workout
GV501.5w43   1994
613.7'1—dc20   94-18268
                        CIP

Workman books are available at special discounts when purchased in bulk for premiums and sales promotions as well as for fundraising or educational use. Special editions or book excerpts can also be created to specification. For details, contact the Special Sales Director at the address below.

Workman Publishing Company, Inc.
708 Broadway,
New York, NY 10003

With the cooperation of Graymont Enterprises, Inc.

Manufactured in the United States of America
First printing December 1994

10 9 8 7 6 5 4 3 2 1

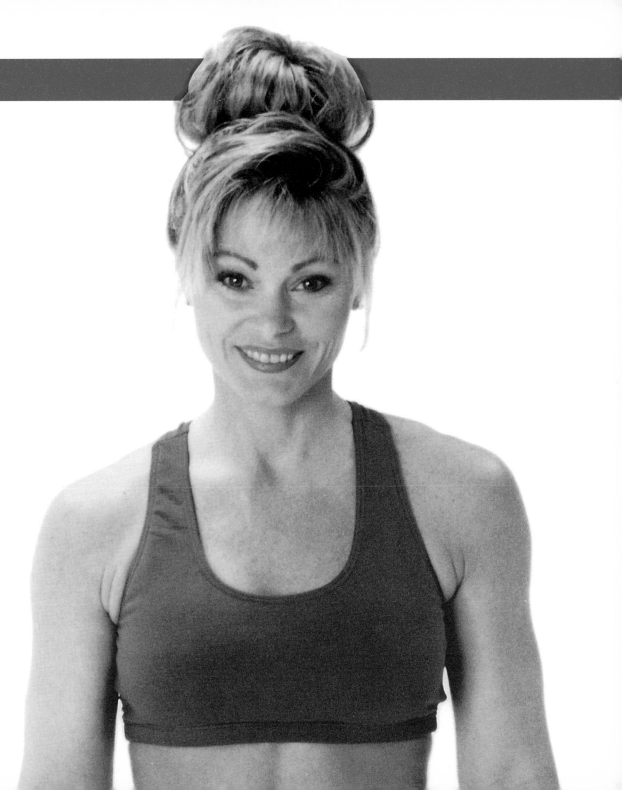

DEDICATION

This book is dedicated to the Physical Education Department at California State University, Chico, especially Dr. William W. Colvin, Dr. Beverly A. Wadsworth, Dr. Robert F. Russ, Dr. Shirley Smith, Dr. Rex R. Grossart, Dr. Thomas Fahey, and Dr. G. David Swanson. The knowledge, guidance, support you have given your students has helped me and so many others to pass on the wisdom. You truly are the real educators of fitness.

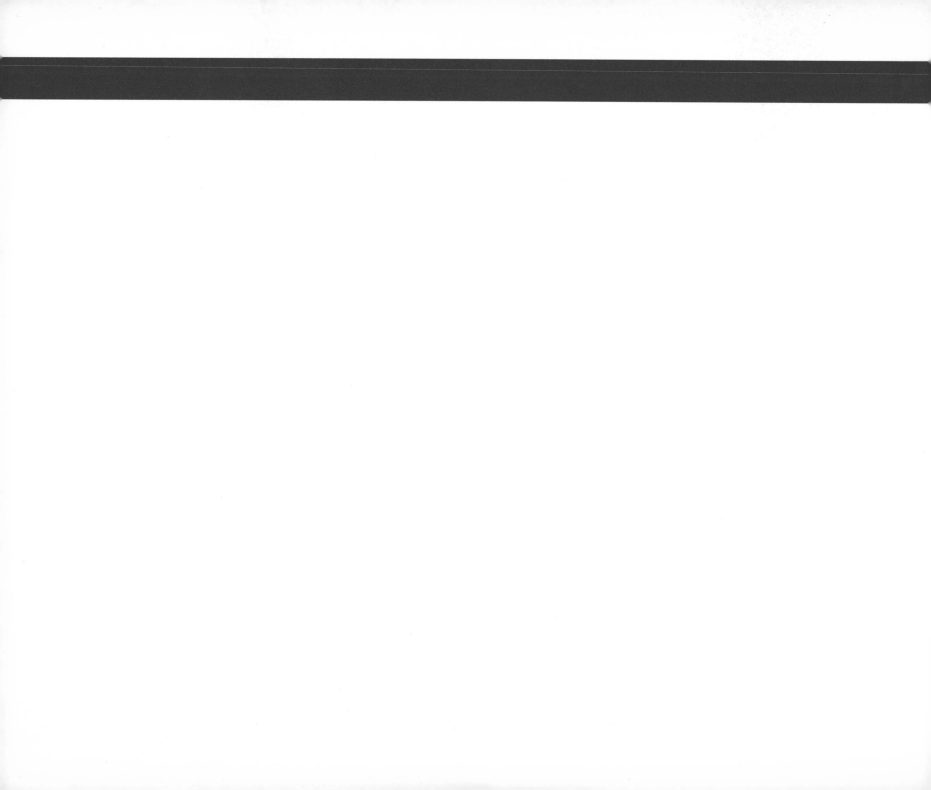

ACKNOWLEDGMENTS

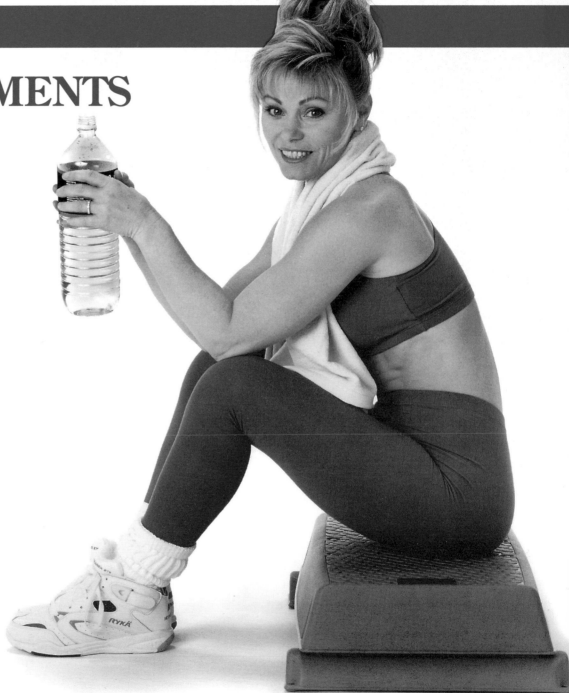

I would like to thank the people who have inspired, supported, and motivated me in completing *Step Up Fitness*. Thanks to Megan Ring, Mindy Marinos, Lori Pawlicki, and the entire staff of Webb International for helping to keep this project going when I was so busy with other projects. Thanks too, to Gin Miller and Reebok for taking step to the public. Thanks to Peter and Lorna Francis for being a moving force in exercise safety. Also, thanks to the editors and staff of Workman Publishing Company for always having a fun and creative approach to all of their books—you're the best in the business! And thanks to Paul Chason, my husband, best friend, and bright light in everything I do—thank you for your love and support.

CONTENTS

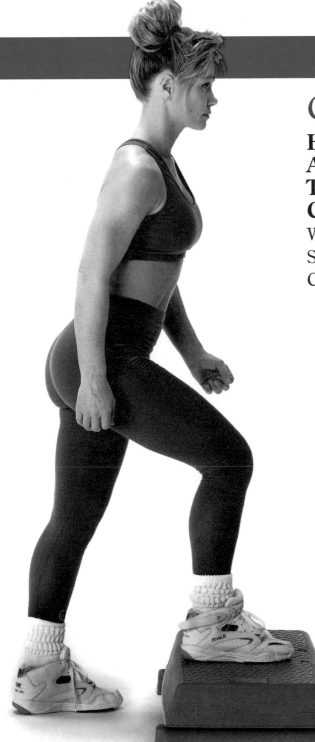

Chapter 3

BEFORE AND AFTER STEPPING: THE WARM-UP AND COOL-DOWN

Chapter 4

THE STEP PATTERNS

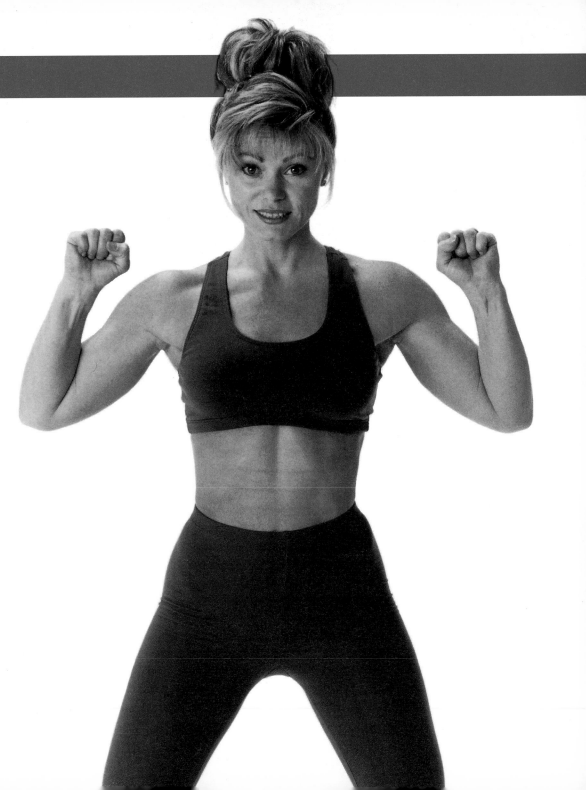

Chapter 7

CHOOSING THE RIGHT STEP UP FITNESS WORKOUT

"Your greatest asset is yourself."

INTRODUCTION

FINDING YOUR INNER SPARK

FINDING YOUR INNER SPARK

One of the unexpected rewards in my years of experience as a fitness trainer has been the opportunity to meet some of the most upbeat, positive people you can imagine. On the outside, they're not much different from anyone you'd bump into at a mall on a busy Saturday afternoon. They're women and men, young people and mature adults, of every size and shape. What makes them different is an inner spark, a recognizable glow of vitality, that says they're onto something special. I can recognize it in an instant.

The "secret" that these wonderful, alive people share is the knowledge that they're in charge of their health and well-being. They know that the choice of fitness over fatness, health over heartbreak (and I mean heartbreak, as in attack), and sanity over "So what?" is theirs and theirs alone. They've learned that health, vitality, and a fruitful, long life are realistic goals that can be achieved through a sensible program of efficient exercise.

If you already know or have the "secret," or you've finally made up your mind to learn it once and for all, I can teach you an easy-to-do exercise program that will increase your fitness and bring you the many other advantages that come with good health.

Readers who are familiar with my *Original Rubber-Band Workout* know that I developed it when I realized that most people who are serious about improving their physical fitness and overall health just don't have the time for an organized program in their daily routine. I knew that not everyone who wants to be fit and trim has access to a gym, a swimming pool, a running track, exercise machines, weights, or the other equipment associated with regular exercise and fitness programs. As a professional who works hard to keep fit and stay on the leading edge of the science of strength training and aerobic exercise, I knew that only a few people who practice a fitness program or who want to begin one have personal trainers.

That meant that there were thousands of people with the best intentions to improve themselves but with no easy, direct way to do it. The answer was my *Original Rubber-Band Workout*, a simple, do-it-in-the-privacy-of-wherever-you-are resistance exercise routine for toning and strengthening all the body's muscles and muscle groups. But there was still something missing.

A convenient program combining cardiovascular fitness with strength training that can be done virtually anywhere, at any time, would be perfect. A program like that would take into account the fact that most people who want control of their physical health and fitness are also active in other areas of their lives. They simply don't have the time to do everything they have to do or want to do the way they would like to. The ideal program would give them—you—the option to train in a self-regulated way that would assure the best use of time and energy to get maximum results.

So here it is. *Tamilee Webb's Step Up Fitness Workout* is based on stepping—a simple routine that fulfills the first requirement of a complete exercise program—cardiovascular fitness.

Basic stepping, as an exercise routine, is a lot like climbing stairs the way little children do, with both feet stopping at each step. The difference is that the stair climber steps to the next step; the stepper returns to the floor. In the basic stepping routine, the stepper places one foot on a low step, steps up, places the other foot on the step, returns the first foot to the floor, and then returns the second. The routine is repeated for a set period of time.

But basic stepping, by itself, isn't enough to qualify as an ideal exercise program. There is a second requirement to a complete exercise program. What is needed is a carefully balanced stepping routine that incorporates muscle-toning exercises of the upper and lower body. Only then can a stepping program be Step Training, the program presented in this book. Step Training is a fully developed combination of stepping routines and muscle-toning moves carefully organized into a progressive program. My Step Training program allows anyone—from absolute beginners to athletes in top shape—to work out privately, at their own pace and on their own schedule, to reach and maintain peak performance.

I knew I had something special and I believe you will, too, once you see what Step Training can do for you. Step Training is the perfect exercise for complete upper- and lower-body conditioning, and meets all the needs of a personal program of fitness and health for our times. It's effective, efficient, quick, convenient—and inexpensive. Step Training is fully aerobic, so you'll gain energy, lose weight, and stay fit. You don't have to go to a gym. And you don't even have to buy special equipment if you don't want to.

"*Welcome to* STEP UP FITNESS, *my personal program for you to get the most out of exercise. You've already taken the first step!***"**

Exercise Then and Now

It wasn't so long ago that physical activity was taken for granted. Good heart-pumping exercise was built into the ordinary activities of daily life—and there were no alternatives. But a lot of the exercise that used to be built into everyday life has been replaced by technology. The result is that we can do a whole lot more with much less physical effort. But the price we're paying for efficiency is tragic and very personal. A lot of it is measured in medical terms that are becoming too familiar: obesity, heart attacks, low energy, depression—the list is frightening.

What troubles me most are the recent trends that have taken away precious physical activity forever. It's not just the cars, planes, elevators, escalators, and automated machinery that reduce our need to move our muscles on a regular basis. It's the things that sneak into our lives and quietly reduce our need for physical activity. Things like telephones, faxes, shopping from catalogs, TV, and video games. Or giant malls that concentrate what used to be blocks-long shopping districts into immense but compact barns—all in the name of convenience. This convenience has a high price—the price of everyday exercise.

The number of people of all ages who get any significant exercise from their daily routines is diminishing. Today, heart-pumping, deep-breathing physical exercise has to be actively pursued. We have to make a deliberate effort to exercise because if we don't, the natural consequences of inactivity will occur.

I believe that the solution to today's fast-paced, no-exercise lifestyle lies with the same kind of technology that took it away in the first place. Through incredible advances in medicine and physiology, we have learned about how the body works and what it needs to stay healthy. The same knowledge and technology that have taken away the stairs to the sixth floor and replaced them with an elevator have also given us a new understanding of the body's "machinery" and systems. It demystifies diet and nutrition. It tells us exactly how the cardiovascular system works. It instructs us, with documented evidence, about what we should and shouldn't do to our bodies. It provides us with the guidelines for exercise and

Exercise improves self-confidence and self-image.

training that assure us maximum benefit.

We're now able to get the most out of exercise because we understand what exercise is and exactly why we need it. We know that exercise is not just activity. It's structured activity with a purpose. That purpose is better health and happier lives.

Advantages of Exercise

M odern medical research has proved that frequent exercise, done correctly, improves health, fitness, and well-being. It does this in many ways, but virtually all are derived from three basic exercise effects.

1. *Exercise reduces body fat and obesity by using the body's stored fat for energy.*

Exercise is physical activity (work) and requires energy. Your body produces its own energy internally from raw materials (food). If you take in more food than you need, your body stores it as fat, and if you store large quantities of unused fats, you become overweight or obese.

2. *Exercise improves the efficiency of the cardiovascular (heart and circulatory) and cardiopulmonary (heart and lungs) systems by increasing the body's need for oxygen.*

The conversion of food to energy is a complex chemical process that depends on oxygen. Your body has to have an ample, constant supply of oxygen to produce energy.

Your body's cells produce energy when sugars and other substances are carried to the cells in the blood and are "burned" when they combine with oxygen. The result is energy and waste products. This cellular conversion of food to energy is more efficient when there's plenty of oxygen, similar to the way the fire in a fireplace burns hotter and brighter when the draft is wide open. The more oxygen you get to the cells, the more efficient the conversion and the more energy you have.

But that's just part of the process. Energy production is also affected by how much energy you need. It's a supply-and-demand situation. The more work (exercise) you do, the more energy you need to do it. When you work hard, you increase your demand for oxygen. While there's always a certain level of oxygen in the blood-

Step Training increases physical strength and stamina.

"Whatever specific benefits you receive, exercise will make you healthier and happier!"

stream and body cells, there's not enough to keep on producing energy, and the demand goes up.

When you increase your activity—run out to the mailbox or climb stairs faster than normal, for example—you increase the demand for oxygen. To supply it, your heart has to pump harder, your lungs have to exchange oxygen and wastes faster, and your vascular system has to transport blood more quickly.

The benefit of increased activity is that your body responds by improving its efficiency. When you place a regular, continued demand on your body by working or exercising hard, your heart, lungs, and vascular system become stronger and better at doing what they do.

3. Exercise improves your psychological and emotional health.

Studies show that moderately intense to intense exercise raises the blood levels of a number of hormones (adrenaline and endorphins) that are associated with feelings of well-being and even euphoria. You're probably familiar with the overall good feeling you're left with after a workout. You feel up, alive, filled with energy. There's a reason. It's more than just feeling good about doing something beneficial for your body. There is a biochemical component of exercise that has a direct psychological effect. You just feel better.

When you put it all together—weight control, improved health, feeling good—you can see how proper exercise can improve your whole person, from head to toe, inside and out.

Revitalize Yourself

Start a well-balanced exercise program now and you can soon expect the following benefits:

• Losing and controlling weight will be easier.

• Your sex life will improve.

• Self-image and self-confidence will improve.

• Personal energy, physical strength, and stamina will increase.

• Stopping smoking will be easier and relapses will be more preventable.

• Stress will be reduced and relaxation will be easier to achieve.

• Muscles will be toned and shaped.

• Sleep will be facilitated.

• Overall body flexibility and joint mobility will increase.

• General health will improve, reducing the chance or probability of illness.

Times Have Changed

Years ago, exercise wasn't very sophisticated because not a whole lot was known about human physiology and the effects of different kinds of exercise on the body. Most people associated exercise with guys in sweaty gyms or adolescent boys in front of bedroom mirrors trying to look like Charles Atlas, their version of Arnold Schwarzenegger. For them, exercise had to do with "ups." There were sit-ups, push-ups, chin-ups, leg-ups, among others.

Like most old-fashioned exercise, the "ups" were based on muscle building and muscle toning. There's nothing wrong with that—I advocate muscle toning, too, as you'll see. The problem with most early exercise programs was that they were limited to building up muscles exclusive of cardiovascular fitness.

Dramatic medical research into how the body works was undertaken in the 1950s and 1960s. By the 1970s, the whole concept of physical conditioning was undergoing enormous changes. The need for exercise was seen as important not just for changing how the body looks but for changing and improving how it works.

As various kinds and levels of exercise were examined, researchers discovered that some types of exercise were better than others. One stood out above all the rest as the best exercise for cardiovascular conditioning and fat burning. Called aerobic exercise, it was based on a whole new understanding of basic physiology and its relationship to heart, lung, and vascular function.

What Is Aerobic Exercise?

There are two basic kinds of physical exercise, aerobic and anaerobic. Both are beneficial. Both use energy and burn fat. Aerobic exercise needs a high volume of oxygen in order to produce the right amount of energy for the activity, whereas anaerobic exercise utilizes the oxygen already in the body's cells and tissues. In other words, your heart works harder and you breathe faster when performing aerobic exercise. You won't find yourself as out of breath doing an anaerobic exercise. Here's why.

The old-fashioned exercises—the "ups" and their related muscle-building cousins—are all anaerobic exercises. *Anaerobic* means "without oxygen." The principle effect of anaerobic exercise is to build muscle tissue. Like all work, anaerobic exercise requires oxygen to produce energy and burn fat, but the rate at which the exercise is performed is slow and its physiological demands on the body are limited.

You can shape and tone your muscles by using resistance in the form of hand weights.

"To obtain the best aerobic effect while exercising, keep your heart rate within your target heart rate range for 20 minutes, three times a week."

Heart Rates

Aerobic training is designed to maximize your cardiopulmonary efficiency. It does this by forcing your heart and lungs to work slightly below your maximum capacity over a prescribed period of time. Your less-than-maximum capacity of cardiopulmonary

Anaerobic exercise produces energy by using the oxygen that is present in muscle tissue and blood, which is easily resupplied by normal breathing. That's why you won't find yourself breathing harder. Regular breathing supplies all the oxygen the body needs.

Aerobic means "with oxygen." Aerobic activity needs more oxygen than you have in your body, and if you want to keep exercising, you need to get more oxygen. If you're running, for example, you first use up the oxygen already in your body, so your breathing at the start of your run is normal. Soon you create a deficit; your reserves get used up and you need more oxygen. When your body's oxygen levels are low, you start breathing harder.

When you exercise vigorously and use up your body's oxygen reserves, your cardiovascular and cardiopulmonary systems compensate by working harder. You breathe deeper and your rate of breathing increases.

At the same time, your heart pumps faster to move the freshly oxygenated blood throughout your body. This kind of exercise is *high-intensity* exercise.

Now, here's the brilliance of your body's marvelous physiological "engineering": If you continue to exercise at your increased level of activity, forcing your heart and lungs to work hard for about 20 minutes, three times a week, you will condition them to handle the increased demand automatically. In a relatively short time, your body's overall efficiency increases. Your lung capacity increases so more air can enter. The strength of your heart muscle increases. Your heart "learns" to pump more blood with fewer strokes. Your lungs "learn" to oxygenate more blood with fewer breaths. Your vascular system "learns" to transport more blood with less effort. And, as long as you continue your weekly routine, they won't "forget." You stay in great cardiovascular shape.

HEART RATES AND TARGET ZONES		
AGE	MAXIMUM RATE (heartbeats per minute)	TARGET RANGE (heartbeats per minute)
20–24	200	120–150
25–29	195	117–146
30–34	190	114–142
35–39	185	111–139
40–44	180	108–135
45–49	175	105–131
50–54	170	102–127
55–59	165	99–123
60–64	160	96–120
65–69	155	93–116
70 and over	150	90–113

efficiency is called your target heart rate, and it can be calculated. Your calculated target heart rate is based on your actual heart rate, which is measured by taking your pulse.

To take your pulse, place two fingertips lightly on the inside of your wrist beneath the thumb of your opposite hand or in the depression next to your windpipe in your neck. Count the number of pulses for 10 seconds and multiply that by 6 to determine the approximate number of times your heart beats per minute. At rest, an average, normal person's heart beats about 70 times a minute. Your own rate may be noticeably different because the normal heart rate range varies for men, women, and age. The best time to take your resting heart rate is just after you wake up, before you get out of bed, because any activity raises the rate.

The rate at which your heart pumps blood when you are working very hard is your maximum heart rate. To calculate your maximum heart rate, subtract your age from 220. For example, if you are 35 years old, 220 − 35 = 185; your maximum heart rate is 185 beats per minute. *Do not exceed your maximum heart rate when exercising* (see the chart).

Research shows that cardiopulmonary conditioning, or aerobic effect, is most productive when you exercise within a

Heart Rate Review

Here's a quick review for calculating heart rates and figuring out your own target heart-rate range:

- Resting heart rate: While at rest, take your pulse for 10 seconds and multiply by 6.

- Maximum heart rate: See the chart on the facing page, or subtract your age from 220.

- Target heart-rate range: Multiply your maximum heart rate by .60 for the low end of the range and by .75 for the high end, or see the chart on the facing page.

percentage range of your maximum heart rate. If you've never exercised before, start off between 50% and 60%. If you have exercised before, but are out of shape, work out between 65% and 70%. And if you're in shape, the range I suggest is between 55% and 90%, the range recommended by the American College of Sports Medicine. This is the *target heart-rate range*.

To determine your target heart-rate range, first calculate your maxi-

mum heart rate or get it from the chart Multiply that number first by .60 and again by .75. For example, a 35-year-old's target heart-rate range would be between 111 and 139 beats per minute ($185 \times .60 = 111$; $185 \times .75 = 139$). For cardiovascular conditioning to occur, that person would have to maintain a heart rate between 111 and 139 beats per minute during three 20-minute exercise periods per week.

A simple way to estimate your target heart rate while exercising to carry on a normal conversation. If you can talk, it's a good indication that you aren't overtaxing your lungs or heart.

Count the number of pulses for 10 seconds and multiply by 6 to determine the approximate number of times your heart beats in a minute.

"There is no such thing as a perfect body. But you can always improve the one you have."

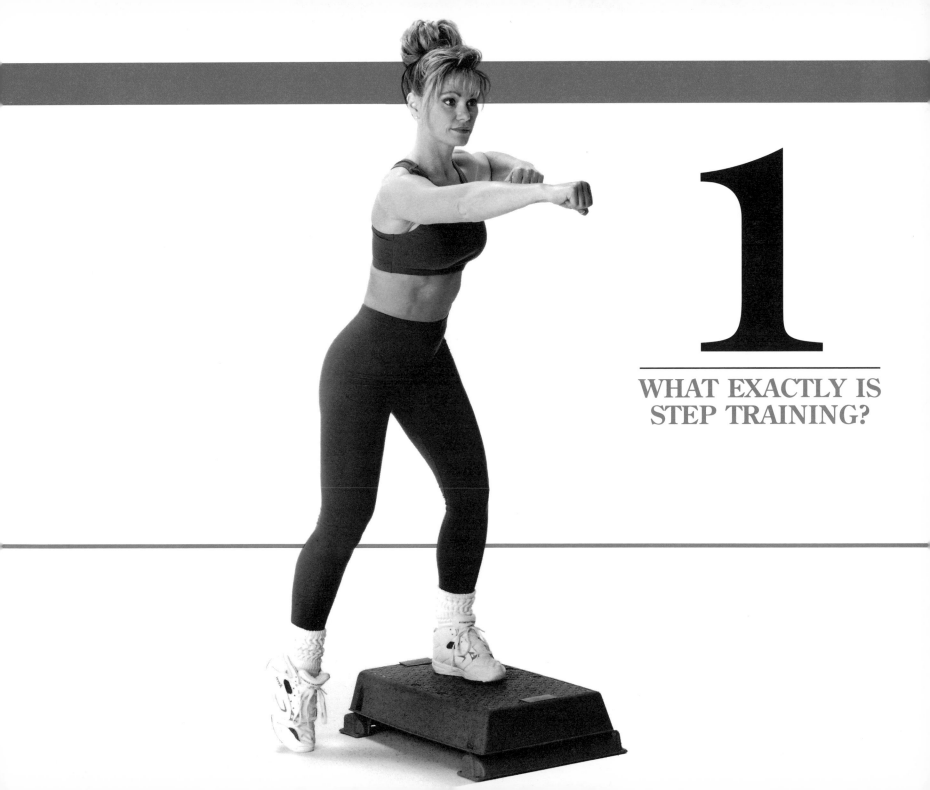

1

WHAT EXACTLY IS STEP TRAINING?

CHAPTER 1

WHAT EXACTLY IS STEP TRAINING?

Step Training is a high-intensity, low-impact, progressive, aerobic body conditioning program. You rhythmically step on and off a low, fixed platform while simultaneously moving your upper body in specific muscle-toning motions. The combined effect is that your whole body and all its major muscle groups get a workout at the same time.

Is Step Training Safe?

First things first: Be sure to check with your physician before starting any exercise program.

Step Training is a low-impact exercise—one foot is in contact with the floor or the step at all times—so there is virtually no major stress on the legs, knees, or lower back.

The degree of impact associated with

Step Training elevates your personal energy.

different kinds of exercise can indicate the level of stress. Running is a high-impact exercise. At each step you hit the ground with your full weight on one foot, over and over, stressing muscles, bones, and joints. Prolonged high-impact activity can produce nasty consequences like shin splints and muscle and joint pain. If treated, these ills are temporary. But permanent damage to connecting tissue in the joints and spine can occur if the activity is not closely monitored.

Roller skating is a low-impact exercise. There is some impact with each stride, but it is negligible. (Falling down is another matter!) Rowing in a boat or on a stationary machine is a no-impact exercise. Low-impact or no-impact exercise places little or no stress on the musculoskeletal system.

When done at high intensity (where your heart rate pumps faster than 180 beats per-minute), both low-impact and no-impact exercise can work you into a fine sweat. The ideal exercise is one that is low or no impact (to protect vulnerable joints and tissues from damage) and one that is high-intensity (to produce the desired aerobic effect) and burns fat.

Step Training is the ideal example of a *low-impact, high-intensity* workout that produces the aerobic effect. You'll sweat, I assure you. You'll condition your heart and lungs, and you won't rattle your spine.

Is Step Training for Me?

If you avoid aerobic exercise classes because the moves are too dancey, too fast, or require too much jumping up and down, the answer is yes. If you hate the monotony of bicycles, stair masters, and other stationary equipment, the answer is yes. If you're already participating in other forms of training and are looking for a new form of exercise to add variety to your standard routines, the answer is yes. And, most important of all, if you're looking for a fitness program that will deliver all the benefits of aerobic exercise in the shortest period of time, the answer is definitely yes.

Fitness enthusiasts at every level of conditioning, from beginners to advanced athletes, will find a challenge in Step Training because the program is easily adaptable to everyone's individual abilities and goals. You can start as a beginning-level stepper and work your way to the top. If you're already at the top, you can use Step Training to stay super fit and trim.

Can Step Training be this good *and* good for you? You bet it is.

The Payoffs

Step Training helps you achieve the following fitness payoffs:

• You reach and maintain your personal aerobic training level quickly, easily, and safely.

• You shape and tone the muscles of both the upper and lower body, with special emphasis on the buttocks, thighs, and legs.

• You burn calories at a maximum rate (about the same as running at 7 miles per hour).

Step Training Is for All Fitness Levels

When you begin a fitness program, you're generally out of shape. After all, that's the usual reason you begin a program. Unless you've been fit all your life (or it's been so long since you weren't fit that you've forgotten), the thought of starting a program is daunting. You want to get into shape, but because you're out of shape, just thinking about the effort is exhausting. That may be a bit exaggerated, but the point is that starting a program when you're out of condition often requires more energy, endurance, and stamina than you think you have. I've been teaching fitness for a long time, and I can tell you firsthand that the drop-out rate in any program is highest in the beginning.

Step Training is a program that permits entry at virtually any level of condition and works up from there. There is a level for someone just beginning, another for those who are in fair condition, and a top level for those in peak condition. In addition, the two lower levels have the goal of conditioning you to reach the next level, while the top level is challenging enough to keep you there. Even if you happen to stop for a while, Step Training lets you resume at a comfort and condition level you can handle.

"*Your body is the only body you'll ever have—take good care of it.*"

What Kind of Equipment Do I Need? What Do I Wear?

You don't have to buy any special equipment, gear, or clothing to begin Step Training. You can if you want to, of course. Or you can wait until you've learned the steps and body-conditioning moves before investing. Either way the cost is manageable.

If you choose to wait to purchase an adjustable Step Training platform, you can begin stepping with any appropriate step in your home. However, home stair steps aren't designed for training, so make sure the step you select meets the following basic requirements.

The home stair riser (the distance from the floor to the step top) should not be over 12 inches. In fact, if you're just beginning, it should be as low as possible (4–8 inches). However, because the height is fixed, the level of Step Training you can reach will be limited. Also, because you can't straddle them, stair steps don't permit some Step Training moves. One of the advantages of the adjustable Step Training platform is that you can start with the platform set at a minimum 4 inches and raise it as you develop stamina. A stair that is too high may exceed your fitness level and is not recommended.

The stair platform (the surface you step onto) should be big enough for your whole shoe. In Step Training, you place the entire sole of your foot on the platform, not just the toes or balls of the feet, so make sure your whole foot fits on the stair step.

Make sure your step platform is stable and secure.

"*Step Training meets all the goals of ideal exercise. And it's incredibly simple.*"

Platform Particulars

A Step Training platform has several advantages over a home stair step. Portability is the most obvious. You can use a Step Training platform almost anywhere.

With the increasing popularity of stepping, a number of platforms have come onto the market. The standard "club" platform that you find in most health clubs and workout centers is about a foot wide and three feet long. Versions made for the home tend to be shorter. A longer platform lets you use a full range of movement when doing some of the traveling patterns (step patterns where you move right or left), and the more you can move, the more intense your workout. Of course, a shorter platform is easier to store.

The key to any platform you buy is adjustability. Step Training is designed to let you progress to advanced levels of exercise, and one way is to increase step height. If you're a beginner, you'll start with your step set at 4 inches high. It won't be long before you'll find an 8-inch height more comfortable, and if you advance further, you might want to increase the height to 10–12 inches. So buy an adjustable platform, if you can. And be absolutely sure that the platform is stable and secure when the adjusting pieces are added or removed.

There are a number of Step Training platforms available at sporting goods stores, fitness equipment suppliers, and department stores. Prices range from about $30 to $100.

When shopping for a Step-Training platform, see that it has the following features:

Shoes

Because Step Training focuses on footwork, it's very important not only to wear shoes but to wear the right shoes. They're essential for two purposes: They must support your feet and they must provide firm footing. Slipping, particularly

Large enough surface. Both feet should fit on it comfortably.

Strength. The center should support your weight.

Rounded edges. This reduces the possibility of injury in case of a slip or fall.

Adjustability. You should be able to raise or lower the step to match your fitness level. (The platform should be 4 inches high when placed flat on the floor; height is adjusted by adding or remov-ing 2-inch risers.)

Sturdiness. The platform shouldn't wobble or slide on the floor.

when you're in the middle of a vigorous program that has you sweating, is always a possibility. Foot support plus good traction will help prevent slipping. Good support, especially of the arches and ankles, will also help protect against injury. Any shoes you use for stepping should have solid lateral and arch support, and the soles should be smooth so that they don't catch on the step. And always wear absorbent cotton socks to wick away moisture inside your shoes.

As for many specialty activities, shoes are available that are designed specifically for stepping; they take into account the demands this high-energy workout places on your feet. You may want to get a pair at the outset or wait until after you have the routines down. Alternatives to stepping shoes are good-quality cross-training shoes. Avoid running, hiking, and street shoes.

Clothing

What you wear is a matter of personal choice, but it has to make sense, too. As in any aerobic training, you'll be using a lot of energy. That's going to produce heat and sweat as by-products, and both have to have someplace to go.

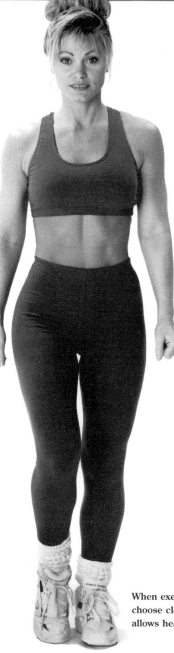

When exercising, choose clothing that allows heat to escape.

Comfort Zone

A simple way to control your comfort level and still make allowances for heat escape is to layer your clothing. Wear a pair of shorts or tights. On top, make the first layer next to your skin an undergarment—a sports bra or supporting top for women, a T-shirt for men. Over that you can wear a loose shirt that slips off easily once you're comfortably warm.

Heat dissipation is especially critical. Overheating can be just plain uncomfortable, but more important, if your body cannot get rid of heat because your clothes act as blankets, prolonged overheating can upset your body's heat-regulating mechanism and lead to cramps, dehydration, and heat exhaustion. Choose clothing that lets built-up heat escape.

Sweat is mostly water, so choose clothing made of absorbent material. In general, whatever you wear, whether it's a warm-up suit, a tank top and tights, or a

T-shirt and shorts, it should be suited to the intensive kind of workout you'll get from Step Training.

Be careful not to wear loose clothing that will get in the way of your activity. Avoid baggy pants or clothes with dangly drawstrings. These could easily tangle up or trip you.

Listen to the Music

Since Step Training is a rhythmic exercise of coordinated moves, it's best to do it to a steady, controlled beat. And, because the objective of Step Training is to raise your heart and breathing rates to aerobically efficient levels and to keep them there for the duration of your workout, the beat should be fairly quick.

The best tempo for Step Training is about 2 beats per second, or 120 beats per minute. A little faster is all right, but 120 beats per minute or slightly slower is better and safer. A faster tempo—135 beats per minute, for example—increases stepping speed to the point that the stepper bounces, which adds unwanted impact stress.

Rather than struggling to keep up a mental tempo, you'll find it a lot easier to keep yourself moving smoothly if you use music. Playing music at the proper tempo is not only the easiest way to keep time as you step, it also motivates and entertains you.

Recorded Step Training tapes at just the right tempo are available at sporting goods, fitness clothing, and exercise equipment stores, or they can be ordered through ads in fitness publications. If you prefer, you can play any recording of your choice that fits the 120-beats-per-minute requirement.

Playing music while you work out is not only entertaining, it can help you keep up the pace too.

"*Music can make you feel good, clothes can make you look good, but it's up to you to feel and look good with or without them.*"

"The secret to reaching and keeping your fitness goals is variety and consistency."

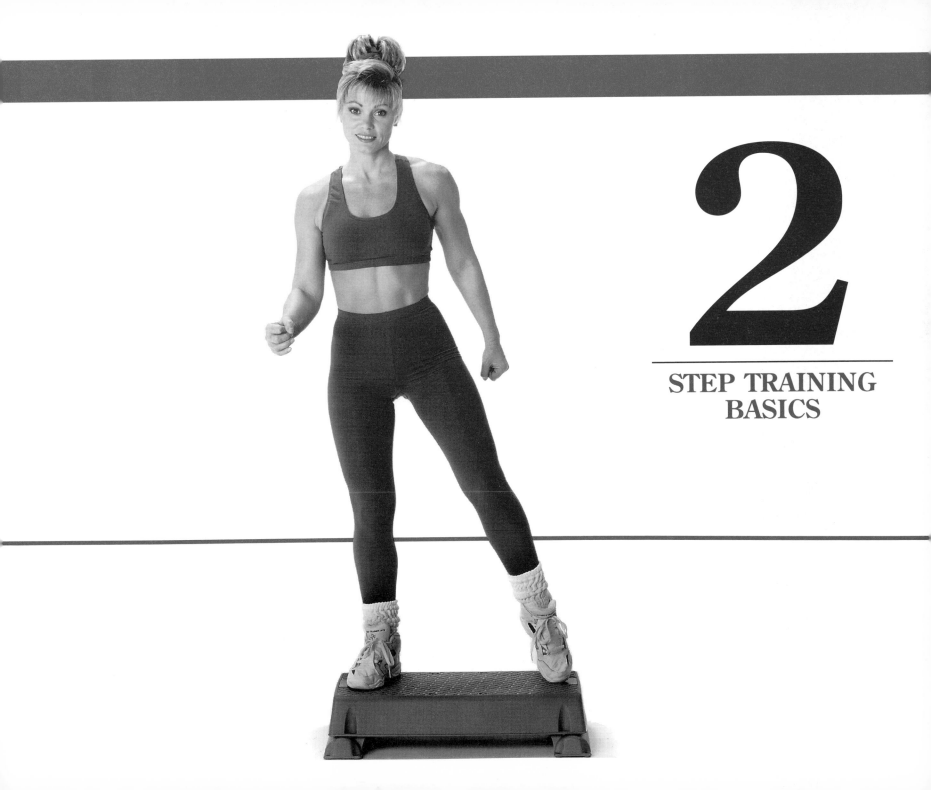

2

STEP TRAINING
BASICS

CHAPTER 2

STEP TRAINING BASICS

While Step Training is a safe, effective form of aerobic exercise, like any fitness program it requires you to pay attention. The more you understand about Step Training, the easier it will be for you to get the maximum benefit from *Step Up Fitness*.

Any fitness program seems a bit daunting when you first learn it. The moves, the beat, and the step-pattern combinations on top of the hard physical work can add up to what seems like a good reason not to bother. Don't let that stop you. It will take a little time to become completely familiar with Step Training, and, yes, it will be hard work. But stay with it. Don't give up. You'll learn the moves sooner than you think, and once you do, you'll really enjoy stepping and even look forward to the exercise.

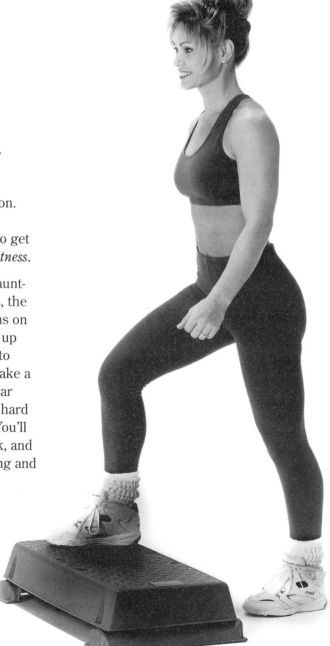

Step Training is safe and effective.

How Frequently Should I Step-Train?

The principles and benefits of aerobic training have been around long enough now that there are accepted standards for frequency (how often) and duration (how long per session) of training. The standards may vary somewhat from program to program and author to author, but they're all in the same range. The American College of Sports Medicine recommends a 20- to 50-minute program of cardiopulmonary conditioning (aerobic exercise) at 55% to 90% of your maximum heart rate—or your target heart rate—two to five times a week.

As you can see, these numbers give you a lot of room for finding a formula that's best for you. They also allow you to start at a lower set of numbers and increase them as your conditioning improves. Once you've reached a comfortable level of training, keep your personal program within these limits for maximum continuing benefit.

Reaching a Target Heart Rate

Your Step Training goal is to exercise in your target heart rate range for a measured period of time. After you've done your warm-up and stretching exercises (Chapter 3), your heart rate will be elevated, but it won't be close to your target rate. (If it is, you may want to check with your physician before beginning the more demanding portion of your workout.)

Once you begin stepping, your heart rate will climb quickly. It will also slow down rapidly when you stop. To be sure that it has returned to normal levels, take your pulse after you've done your cool-down If your heart rate is still high, continue the cooldown, gradually reducing the activity. Or, if you choose, take a short stroll after cooling down. In the beginning, unless you're an experienced aerobic trainer, you won't know what intensity of stepping you need to get you to your target rate and keep you there. After a while, it will be second nature.

To determine the intensity of activity at which you reach your target heart rate, begin by stepping the Basic Right and Basic Left step patterns (pages 44–47). Do the Basic Right step pattern for 1½ minutes and the Basic Left step pattern for 1½ minutes, then stop and take your pulse. Take it quickly, because it will begin to slow down the instant you stop stepping. If your pulse is higher than your target rate, reduce the intensity of stepping. If it's lower, increase the intensity.

To alter your workout intensity, raise or lower your platform, or increase or decrease your arm and upper body movements. The tempo should remain constant.

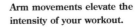

Arm movements elevate the intensity of your workout.

Body Alignment

It is important to keep your body in proper alignment to eliminate the possibility of injury. Take the time to concentrate on making sure your body is in the correct position. Never locking your knees and always keeping your body forward and relaxed gives you the full range of motion and maximizes your effort in Step Training.

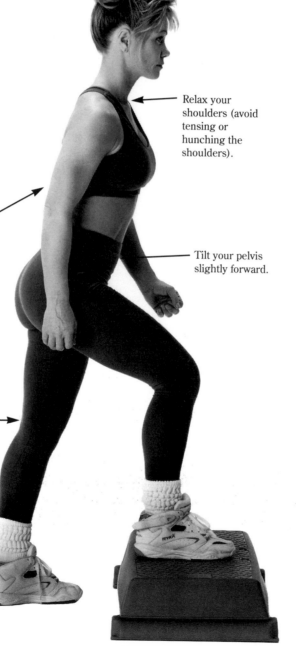

Relax your shoulders (avoid tensing or hunching the shoulders).

Lean forward slightly so that your body is inclined at about 75 to 80 degrees.

Tilt your pelvis slightly forward.

Flex your knees slightly (don't lock them, and don't extend them fully).

Platform Height

The intensity of your Step Training will progress as your ability and stamina improve. A beginning stepper needs a lower platform height than intermediate or advanced steppers. Also, platform height should correspond to the stepper's size. As a general rule, step heights should be selected as follows:

• Choose a 4-inch height if you are a beginning stepper who is new to exercise or pregnant (and then only with your physician's permission).

• Choose a 6-inch height if you are a beginning stepper who exercises on a regular basis.

• Choose an 8-inch height if you are an intermediate stepper, in good shape, who has been stepping for 8 weeks.

• Choose a 10-inch height if you are an advanced stepper.

• Choose a 12-inch height if you are a well-conditioned, tall athlete who has fully mastered stepping.

Feet First

The feet and ankles provide support for your whole body when Step Training. This is reason enough to be conscientious about placing your feet properly. Your feet should always point straight ahead and your weight should be distributed along the whole foot. When you step up on the platform, the entire foot must be on the platform. If your heels hang off, you could twist your ankle or pull a tendon.

Think about how your foot is landing each time you step up or down. Always step ball to heel. Landing on your heel first is jolting to your body and can cause pain and discomfort later. It may seem like a lot to think about, but being methodical when you are learning the basics ensures good habits and the best benefits for the rest of your life.

Once you place your feet accurately, the movement will feel natural and the proper way to step will be automatic. The picture shows some specifics to keep in mind.

Keep your toes pointed straight ahead and your weight distributed along the whole foot.

Place the entire bottom of your foot in contact with the platform.

Always step directly onto the platform center when stepping up.

When stepping down, place the entire bottom of your foot in contact with the floor—ball to heel.

Leg Movement

Your legs move naturally when you're stepping, although foot placement will depend on which step pattern you're doing. You'll see what I mean when I describe each pattern in Chapter 4. In every case, however, do not allow the knee of your base leg to flex so that it extends past your toe. Your knee should always be directly above your ankle. Keep your leg movements natural, though you may exaggerate them slightly, if you choose.

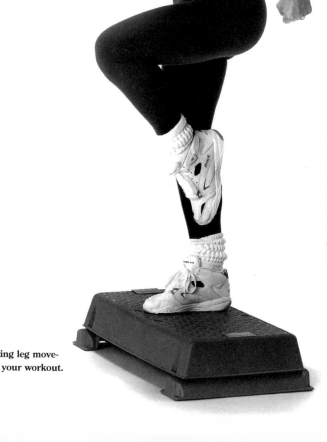

Slightly exaggerating leg movements intensifies your workout.

Arm Movement

Your arms move in a natural swing when you walk or run. When you step forward with one leg, the opposite arm swings forward. This is your body's way of maintaining balance when walking upright. Step Training is just as natural as walking and your arm movements follow the same pattern they do when you walk. However, rather than letting your arms hang at your sides as they do while you are casually walking, you'll be more comfortable if you hold them semiflexed with your hands in a soft fist, the closed palms facing one another. The best way to achieve this position is to imagine that you're carrying a candle in each hand.

Let your arms swing in a natural cadence as you step, or, if you prefer, you can exaggerate the movement to increase the intensity of your workout. All by itself, arm pumping is an excellent workout. While you are a beginner, though, concentrate on the steps. When you feel confident of the steps, you can add the arm movements described in Chapter 5.

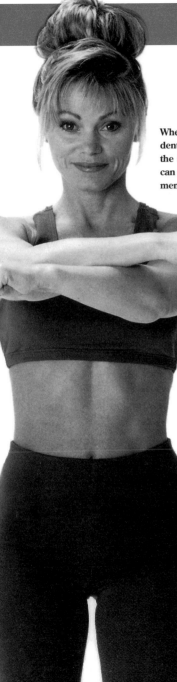

When you feel confident that you know all the step patterns, you can add arm movements.

Safety Tips

Step Training is safe when performed properly. To assure safe, effective workouts, keep the following tips in mind as you enjoy *Step Up Fitness*.

• Get your physician's permission to exercise.

• Pay attention as you train!

• Watch your pulse and breathing rates diligently.

• Before each session, make sure your platform is stable.

• You'll sweat a lot, so drink plenty of liquids before, during, and after a workout.

• To avoid slipping, keep a towel nearby to wipe any perspiration off the platform.

• Step onto the center of the platform when stepping up; when stepping off, step back, not forward off the step, landing close to the platform.

• Place the sole of your foot firmly on the platform with each step up; don't let your toes or heels hang over the edge.

• Check your foot placement on the platform every few seconds to make sure you're landing correctly.

"Exercise can improve your whole person from head to toe, inside and out."

"Be patient! The rewards of exercise are great."

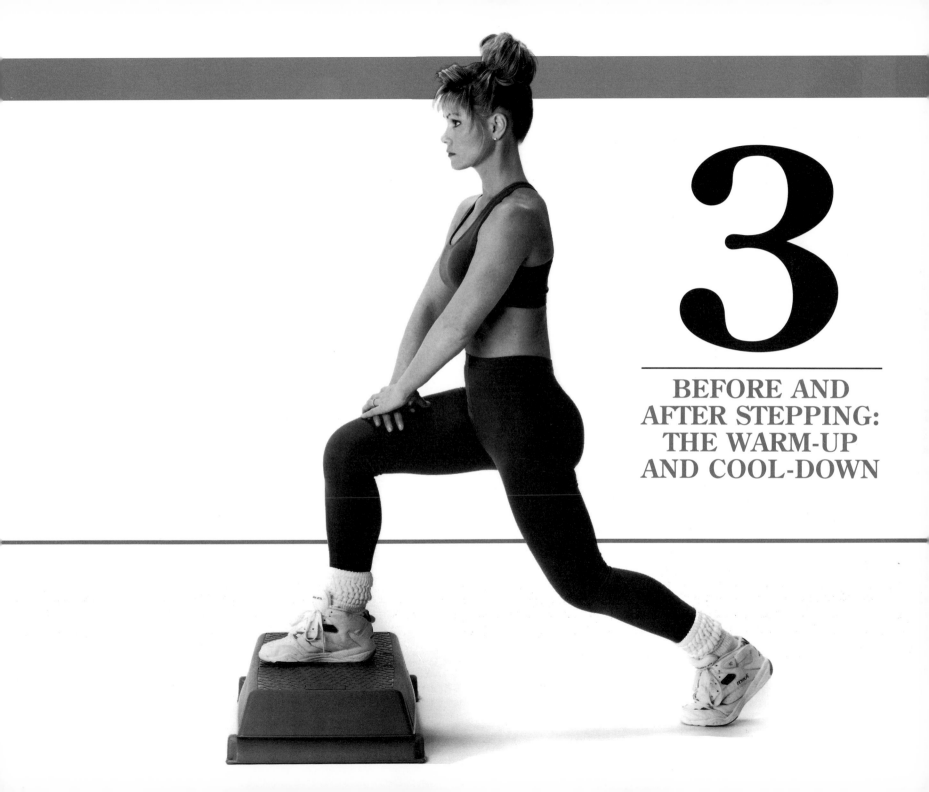

3

BEFORE AND AFTER STEPPING: THE WARM-UP AND COOL-DOWN

CHAPTER 3

BEFORE AND AFTER STEPPING: The Warm-Up and Cool-Down

As in all good exercise programs, each one of your Step Training workouts will have a beginning, a middle, and an end. Because each part leads to the next and all are important to your overall workout, no parts should be skipped. The warm-up and cool-down exercises are exactly the same, though they serve different functions. The warm-up period, for example, prepares your body for the vigorous aerobic portion of the workout. It begins to raise your heart rate and "loosen" your muscles and connective tissues to help protect you against injury. Also, warming up gets you into a good mind-set for working out. Similarly, the cool-down and stretch period after an invigorating exercise is an essential stage in getting the most from your workout.

Stretching loosens muscles and primes you for vigorous exercise.

Slowing down your heart rate and breathing rate along with stretching your muscles prevents pain and stiffness as it allows your systems to gradually return to normal.

I can't emphasize enough the importance of properly warming up, stretching, and cooling down as a part of any program, because they are the keys to avoiding injury and getting the most from your workout.

The body's soft tissues—muscles, tendons, and ligaments—are made of fibers that can stretch and contract. The older we get, the less supple they are. These tissues tend to feel "tight" when unused for a period of time, and as anyone who has overtaxed themselves will tell you, they can get painfully stiff after rigorous use when you're out of condition. The feeling of tightness is real. Tissues that aren't periodically stretched contract. Sudden use stretches them or even tears them, resulting in pain. This type of injury is common in any active sport involving major limb movement. All serious athletes begin every practice and competition with a complete warm-up routine. Warming up and stretching prepares muscles and tissues for the demands of exercise.

Total Workout

Each Step Training workout includes three segments. The three main sections are:

- *Warm-up and stretch*
This elevates heart rate and limbers up your body in preparation for active exercise.

- *Step Training*
Stepping combined with body sculpting conditions your whole body.

- *Cool-down and stretch*
This gradually slows down heart rate and allows your body to return to normal.

Warming Up

The gradual movements of warming up and stretching slowly elevate your heart rate, increase your circulation, speed up your breathing, and begin to raise your body temperature so that when you begin stepping vigorously, your whole body and all its systems are prepared. When you've finished the Step Training workout, the cooling down and stretching period allows your body systems to gradually return to normal.

Each of your warm-up periods should be 5 to 8 minutes long including stretches. Your movements should be bold and rhythmic and your breathing deep and relaxed. Begin slowly and work up to a faster tempo. Your first moves can even be cautious, as if you were testing your muscles and joints (especially if you're stiff or haven't worked out in a while). After you feel more confident, you can extend warm-up movements to their full range.

If you have a favorite warm-up routine that you've followed in other programs, use it. Make sure it includes arm and upper-body moves, however, because as you'll see, Step Training is a complete program of upper- and lower-body conditioning. Your warm-up should get every part of your body—from your head to your toes—ready to go to work.

The gradual movements of stretching and warming up slowly elevate your heart rate.

Here's the warm-up sequence I recommend. You'll find that after a few repetitions, this warm-up sequence will come naturally.

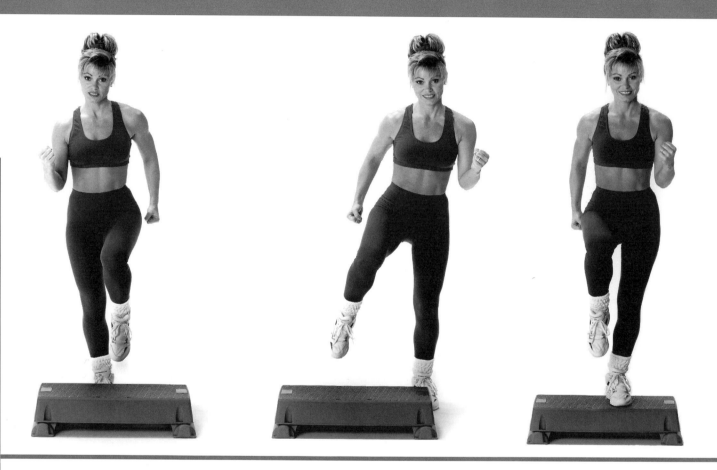

Revving Up

- Stand on the floor facing the platform.

- Start with right leg.

- Do each warm-up exercise for a count of 8.

- When you have completed each of the warm-up exercises, repeat the entire sequence 3 times.

Warm-up 1

March in place on the floor for a count of 8 (right + left = 1 count). Gradually raise your knees higher as you march until you strut with your knees coming to just under hip level.

Warm-up 2

Spread your legs and march with your feet about shoulder width apart. This is called the Wide Step. Using the Wide Step, march in place on the floor for a count of 8. Gradually raise your knees higher as in Warm-up 1.

Warm-up 3

Step up on top of the platform with your feet comfortably together and march for a count of 8, gradually raising your knees higher as in warm-up 1.

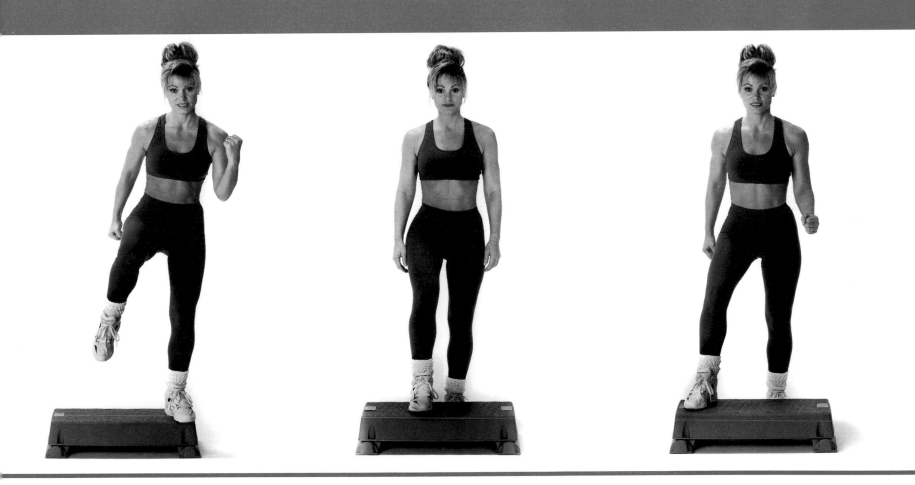

Warm-up 4

Wide Step on top of the platform for a count of 8, gradually raising your knees higher as in Warm-up 1.

Warm-up 5

Step back to the floor and, while marching in place at the same tempo, alternately tap the top center of the platform with your right toe and left toe. Do this step for a count of 8.

Warm-up 6

Still marching in place at the same tempo, alternately tap the right end of the platform with your right toe and the left end of the platform with your left toe for a count of 8.

Stretching

Now that your heart rate is up, it's time to stretch. It is important to warm up before you do any stretching because muscles and tendons stretch more easily when the body temperature is raised.

The stretching portion of your workout prepares you not only physically for the effort of a dynamic workout, it prepares you psychologically as well. Easing into a workout with the extended motions of stretching allows you to get in touch with your body and feel which areas may be stiff or need special attention.

Stretching the muscle fibers prepares them for the intense activity of a workout. "Loose" muscles are more capable of handling the rigors of exercise than "tight" ones. If you don't carefully warm up and stretch, an intense workout could cause muscle cramping, pulled tendons, or torn muscles. New understanding and respect for the importance of stretching has evolved over the past few decades. Thorough warm-up exercises and stretching significantly decreases the chance of injury. Often overlooked or poorly executed in the workout regime, a stretching routine is not only a good idea, it is essential to making your body a well-oiled, balanced, and finely tuned machine, ready to reap the benefits of exercise.

Chest (pectoralis major and minor)

The goal of the following stretching exercises is to lengthen the muscle fibers and keep your muscles and tendons supple and your body balanced and flexible. This is achieved by taking your time and completing each stretch firmly and gently. And don't forget to breathe. Your tissues need all the oxygen they can get as they loosen up. By leaning deliberately into a stretch and holding it for 10–30 seconds, you will actually be elongating the muscle fibers. The musle fibers move a lot like rubber bands. You can stretch a rubber band for a great length if you stretch gently, but if you are too aggressive, you can snap or tear it. Similarly, a muscle stretched too far can tear and leave you in agony.

Hip flexor (illiopsoas)

Front of thigh (quadriceps)

Concentrate on the specific muscle groups when stretching.

Muscle- and connecting-tissue stretches should be small and gentle—not forced at all. Never stretch to the point of pain. Stretch to the point of tightness. If your body sends you a signal of pain, listen to it. It's trying to tell you something. Be very careful to allow tissues to lengthen gradually. Move gracefully and evenly. Avoid bouncing, pumping, or jerking. Each movement should be performed in slow motion. The whole idea behind stretching is to prevent injuries, not create them.

As you begin stretching, you may notice that you don't feel very flexible. Each one of us has a different range of flexibility. The basis of flexibility can be genetic. You may be in terrific shape but not be able to touch your toes. Some people may be flexible in the hip joints but not so flexible in the back. Whatever your range of flexibility is, you can improve it with patience and dedication.

You'll do two stretching sequences in each workout, one in your warm-up and the other in your cool-down at the end of your workout. For both sequences, familiarize yourself with the muscles and muscle groups indicated on these pages and focus on them as you stretch.

Upper back (rhomboids)

Back of thigh (hamstring)

Calf (gastroncinius)

Focused stretching prepares muscles for the demands of exercise.

Stretching It

Because it's possible to overstretch and damage tissue, follow these precautions when stretching:

- Breathe slowly and deeply as you stretch.

- Do not bounce, jerk, or force stretches.

- Stretch at your own pace, paying attention to what you are doing.

- Stretch gently.

- Hold warm-up and cool-down stretches to a count of 30 seconds.

- Stop stretching when you feel pain; don't stretch through it.

If you have a stretching sequence you already use, stay with it, if you like. If not, use the following succession of stretches.

Don't Force It

If you aren't very flexible, be patient, you will be. Never bounce or yank a stretch. Approach each movement firmly and gently. Create a comfortable connection between your muscle and the stretch. You should feel a slight pull. Breathe deeply and stretch just a little further. With gentle persistence, it won't be long before you experience longer and stronger muscles and more flexible joints.

Back of thigh

Place your right foot on the platform. Rest both hands on your left thigh and bend both knees. Bending from the hips, but keeping your back straight, press your hips back and extend your right leg. Your weight should be on your left leg. You'll feel this stretch in the back of your right leg. Hold for 30 seconds. Repeat with the left leg. *Safety Tips:* Don't bounce. Don't lock the knee joint.

Front of thigh

Place your right foot on the platform. Rest your arms on your right thigh. Keeping your weight forward, extend your left leg, slightly bent, behind you. Press your pelvis forward. You'll feel this stretch in the front of your right leg. Hold for 30 seconds. Repeat with the left leg. *Safety Tips:* Keep your knees bent. Don't arch your back.

Calf

Stand with both feet on the platform, knees slightly bent. Then lower one heel off the back of the step and press down. You'll feel the stretch in this calf. Hold for 30 seconds. Repeat with the other leg. *Safety Tips:* Don't bounce. Don't lock your knee joint.

Hip flexor

Place your right foot on the platform, with your knee bent at a 90° angle. Extend your left leg behind you, and balance on the ball of your left foot. Slowly lower your body downward while pressing the hip of the extended leg slightly forward. Feel the stretch in the front of your left hip. Hold for 30 seconds. Repeat with the other leg. *Safety Tip:* Don't bend your knees beyond a 90° angle.

Upper back

Stand with both feet together or with one foot upon the platform for better balance. Reach both arms out in front with hands clasped together. Press and extend your arms forward. Your back should be rounded. Feel the stretch in your upper back. Hold for 30 seconds. *Safety Tip:* Tilt your chin down toward your chest and exhale.

Chest

Stand with both feet together or with one foot up on the platform for better balance. Clasp your hands together behind your back. Extend and lift them up and away from your body. You should feel the stretch across your chest. Hold for 30 seconds. *Safety Tips:* Don't arch your lower back. Don't bend over.

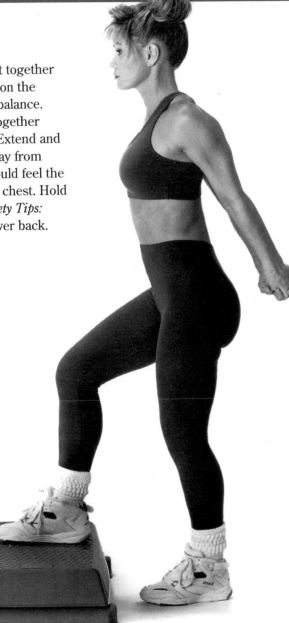

Cooling Down

When you have finished your Step Training workout, it's time to cool down. Cooling down and stretching is just as important as warming up because it lets your body systems gradually return to normal. To suddenly go from a high-intensity workout to a complete standstill would produce an unnecessary shock to your body. This shock is easily avoided by intentionally slowing down and cooling down.

To cool down properly, repeat the entire warm-up sequence three times. Then carefully perform each stretch. Remember to hold each stretch for 30 seconds.

The period immediately following the cool-down is one of unusual well-being and calm. You've finished the workout, you're fully relaxed, and it'll be yours all over again at your next training session. Done properly, exercise is a gift to yourself that keeps on giving.

"All athletes begin and end every practice and competition with a complete stretching routine."

"Tap into the power of your own healthy body."

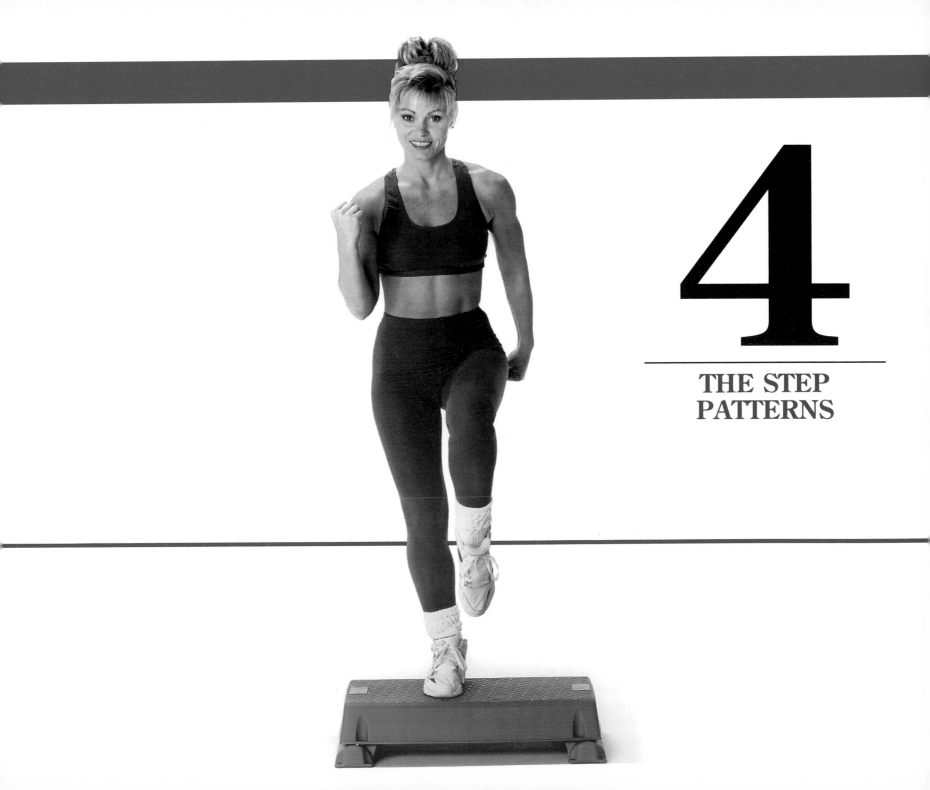

4

THE STEP
PATTERNS

CHAPTER 4

STEP PATTERNS

The first time you watch someone stepping you may find yourself saying, "I can't possibly remember all those moves." But don't worry, Step Training is a lot simpler than it looks. The patterns will seem effortless to you after a short time. It's true that they're a little more involved than the moves in climbing a set of stairs, but I can assure you they're much less complicated than the steps in the merengue. My Step Training workout is designed to move from simple to more complex step patterns. Once you have mastered basic movements, you'll be ready to combine them in the workout that fits your current condition. I describe the various workouts in detail in Chapter 7.

Starting Positions

There are five starting positions from which you may begin a step exercise. This allows for variations in the step patterns themselves and in the workouts. The most common starting position is the front—with the long edge of the platform facing you. Get to know the starting positions and pay attention to which starting

Step Aside

Whichever position you start from, keep these two points in mind:

• From any starting position, both feet should be slightly apart and should face straight ahead. Your toes should be directly in front of your heels.

• Any time you start an exercise with the side of your body facing the step platform, the leg closest to the step should step first.

position a particular pattern begins with. You'll quickly memorize them and they will become instinctive. If you get confused during a specific pattern or in the midst of a workout, you can always go back to the starting position and begin again.

In any starting position, make sure both feet are not too far away from the platform. Feet should be pointing in the same direction, knees slightly bent and chest up. Remember that when you step, you should move smoothly and not bounce—bouncing puts stress on muscles and tendons.

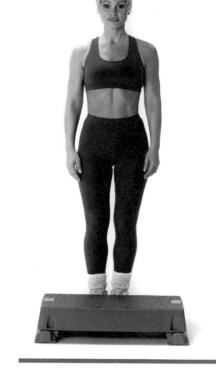

Front In the front starting position, the long edge of the platform is centered in front of you.

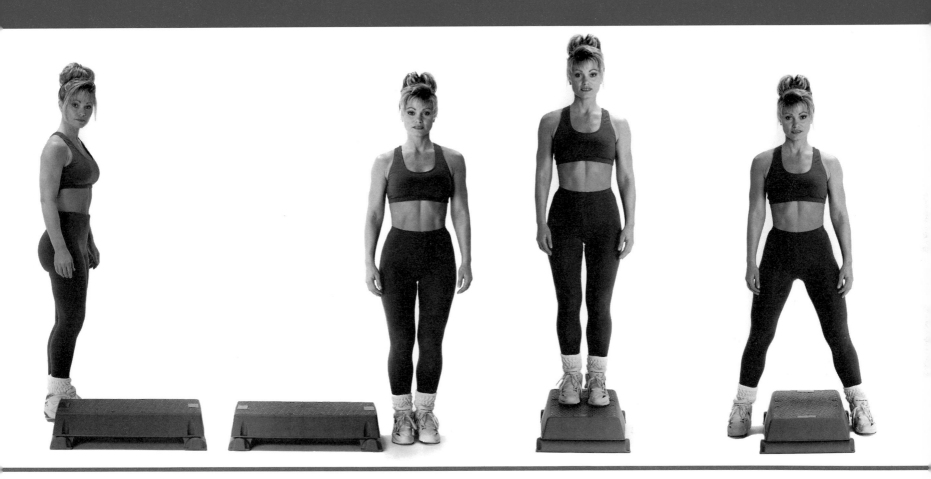

Side In the side starting position, you stand with your side toward the long edge of the platform.

End In the end starting position, the short edge of the platform is to your side.

Top In the top starting position, you stand on top of the platform, with your toes pointing to the short edge and the long edges at your sides.

Straddle In the straddle position, one foot is placed on either side of the long edge of the platform.

A Beat in Time

Now that you're familiar with the starting positions, you're ready for the step patterns themselves. A step pattern is a series of basic stepping movements strung together. Each step pattern is made up of either four or eight of these basic stepping movements or beats. Beats make up a pattern and patterns make up a workout.

All the workouts consist of step patterns. It's these basic patterns that you will learn first. The easiest way to learn a pattern is to go through it step by step or beat by beat—the way you do when learning a dance step. You don't have to use music at this point, but you will learn the steps and the patterns in terms of beats.

All step patterns are based on a natural rhythm. The steps will be easier to learn if you keep in mind that each step in a pattern is one beat and that each pattern is made up of either four or eight beats. Each photograph represents a movement which corresponds to a numbered beat in the step pattern. You can see the numbers under each movement followed by a complete description of each step.

Concentrate on each step within the pattern. Once you've done a few repetitions, count the beat out loud again without music. That way you can slow down the beat to let your feet catch up. After you feel confident with the pattern, add the music of your choice. Remember, 120 beats per minute is ideal—2 beats per second. Of course, you can start slower if you want to until you're comfortable. Then you can work up to 120 beats later.

Music is a great way to keep you going. It's fun and it helps you to keep your movements steady and constant. The energy of a fast-moving song can keep your enthusiasm high and make the whole process of getting in shape exhilarating.

In this chapter, each step pattern is presented so that it can be easily followed by the beginning or the advanced stepper. The patterns are shown without specific arm movements. Arm movements are described in Chapter 5 and can be added once you are adept at the step patterns.

Learning the step patterns is easier than learning to dance.

Step Stats

For each step pattern, look for the corresponding chart that gives you the following information:

- Number of beats

- Basic starting position

- Number of repetitions recommended for each pattern

The Step Stats box gives you information specific to the particular pattern. It shows the number of beats in the pattern, the starting position, and the number of times to repeat the pattern.

Before you begin a pattern, read the directions carefully, including all safety tips. Familiarize yourself with the steps or beats involved in the pattern. Concentrate on doing each step accurately and follow the photographs as closely as possible. If you are learning these patterns for the first time, it is crucial to have correct body alignment and form for maximum exercise effectiveness and to avoid the possibility of injury. Move smoothly and rhythmically, let your arms swing naturally, and make sure your feet are always placed securely on the platform.

There are 17 step patterns described in the following pages. Each step pattern has a name such as Basic Right or Wide Step. And each pattern has a specific number of steps or beats. After you learn these step patterns individually, you will string the separate patterns together to create a total body workout that is perfectly suited to you. Practice each step pattern separately until you know it, then move on to the next pattern. Don't be discouraged if you feel awkward at first. Soon you'll be stepping up to fitness and having fun too!

Proper body alignment is important for getting the most out of your workout and for avoiding injury.

"Ten minutes is better than no minutes. Twenty minutes is better than 10 minutes. And 30 minutes a day of physical exercise is just right."

BASIC RIGHT

This is the most basic step pattern in any workout. Always remember to start off with your right foot. Step up on the platform with your right, and step down from the platform with your right.

Step Stats

- 4 beats
- Starting position: Front
- Repetitions: 8 (32 beats)

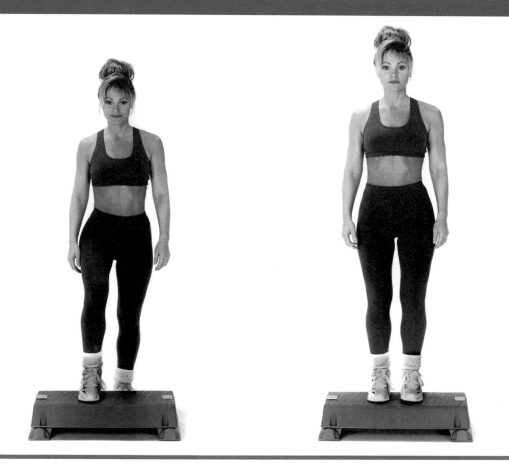

1 From the front starting position, lift your RIGHT foot and place it squarely on the platform, ball of foot to heel. Keep your arms relaxed and your chest lifted.

2 Step up with your LEFT foot, ball to heel, so that you're standing with both feet flat on the top of the platform, your weight equally distributed between them.

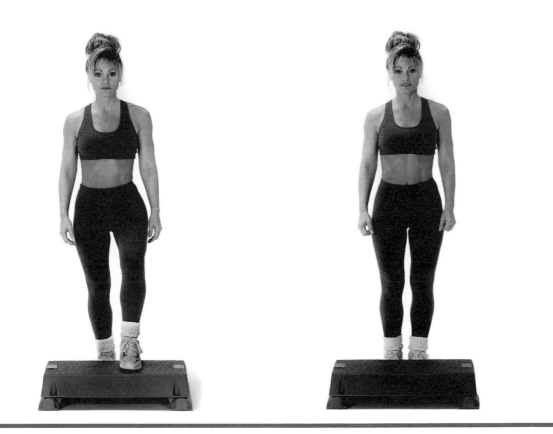

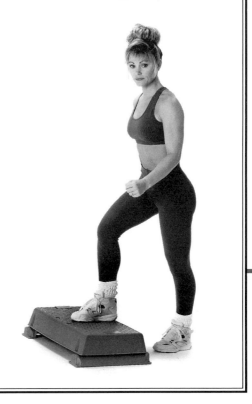

DON'T LOCK UP

Whenever you step down, always keep your knees slightly bent. Locking your knees places strain on the tendons and ligaments and could cause pain and serious damage.

3 Lift your RIGHT foot from the platform and step back to the floor, ball to heel.

4 Lift your LEFT foot from the platform and return it to the floor, ball to heel. You should be in the same position as when you started, with weight equally distributed between both feet.

BASIC LEFT

This is exactly the same pattern as the Basic Right, except that you always lead off with your left foot. Step up with your left and step down with your left.

Step Stats

- 4 beats
- Starting position: Front
- Repetitions: 8 (32 beats)

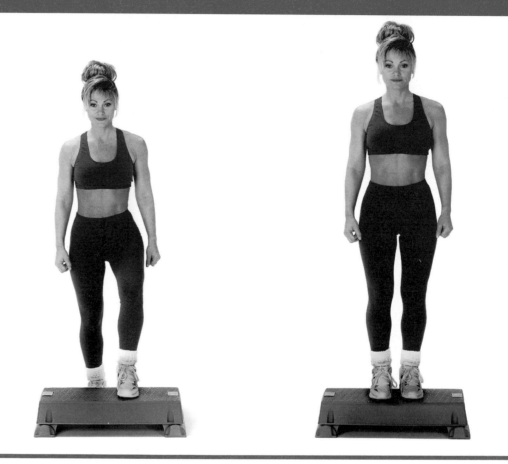

1 From the front starting position, lift your LEFT foot and place it squarely on the platform, ball to heel. Your arms should be relaxed and your chest lifted.

2 Step up with your RIGHT foot, ball to heel so that you're standing with both feet flat on the top of the platform, your weight equally distributed between them.

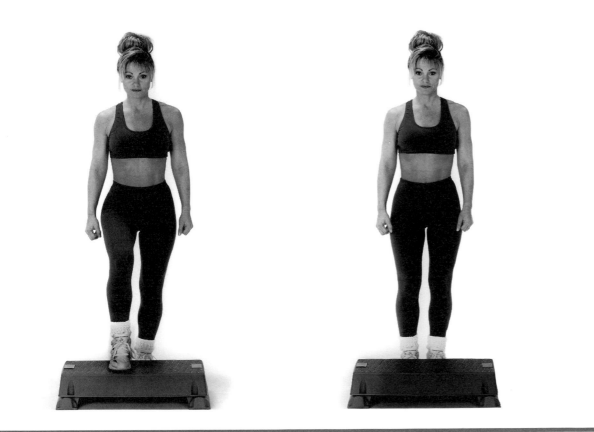

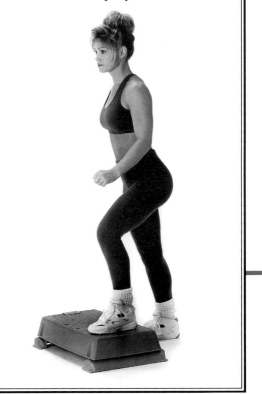

STANDING TALL

When stepping up on the platform, keep your weight forward, your head up, and your abdomen tucked in. Good posture and alignment prevents soreness and injury.

3 Lift your LEFT foot from the platform and step back to the floor, ball to heel.

4 Lift your RIGHT foot from the platform and return it to the floor, ball to heel. You should be in the same position you were when you started, with your weight equally distributed between both feet.

WIDE STEP

The wide step is similar to the Basic Right in movement, but in this pattern, you step wide on the platform. Pretend there is a big hole in the center of the platform.

Step Stats

- 4 beats
- Starting position: Front
- Repetitions: 8 (32 beats)

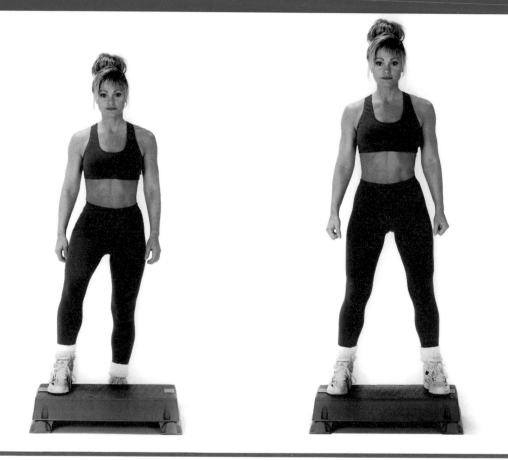

1 From the front starting position, lift your RIGHT foot and place it squarely on the RIGHT end of the platform, ball to heel. Keep your shoulders square, your back straight, and your toes pointed straight ahead.

2 Step up with your LEFT foot, ball to heel, placing it on the LEFT end of the platform so that you're standing with both feet flat and wide apart on the top of the platform. Your weight should be equally distributed.

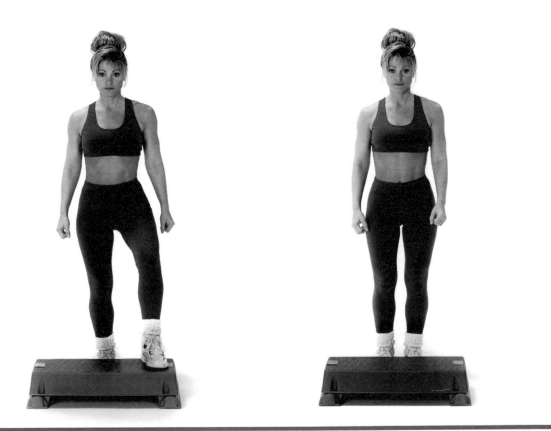

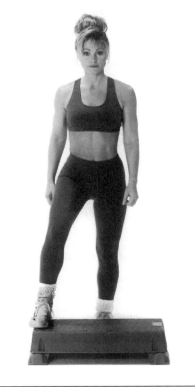

WATCH YOUR STEP!

Never step so wide that your feet hang off any edge of the platform. To avoid ankle injuries, every part of your foot should be on the step. Check your foot placement every once in a while to make sure.

3 Lift your RIGHT foot and step back to the floor behind the center of the platform, ball to heel.

4 Lift your LEFT foot and bring it back to the floor, next to your right foot. You should be in the same position you were in when you started, with your weight equally distributed between both feet.

ALTERNATING TAP DOWN

This is the first pattern in which there are eight beats. You will alternately tap your right and left toe on the floor on the fourth and eighth beats.

Step Stats

- 8 beats
- Starting position: Front
- Repetitions: 4 (32 beats)

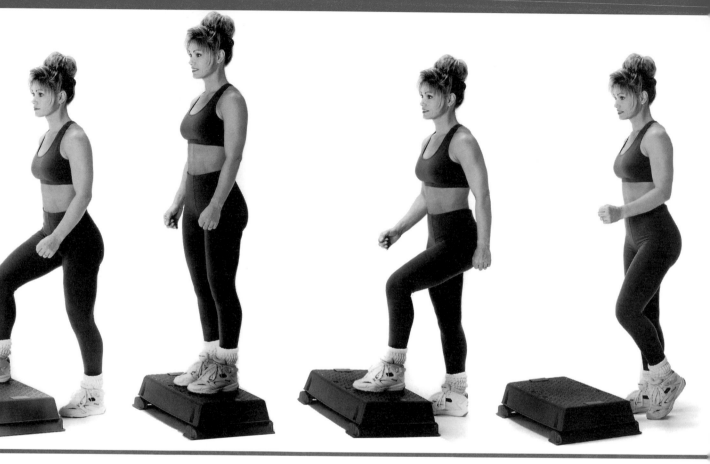

1 From the front starting position, lift your RIGHT foot and step squarely on the platform, near the center, ball to heel. Make sure your heel is not hanging off the edge.

2 Step up with your LEFT foot, ball to heel, so that you're standing on the top of the platform with both feet next to each other. Your weight should be equally distributed between them.

3 Lift your RIGHT foot and step back to the floor. Be careful not to lock your knees.

4 Lift your LEFT foot and TAP DOWN with your LEFT toe on the floor about 6 inches from your right foot. Don't step down, just tap.

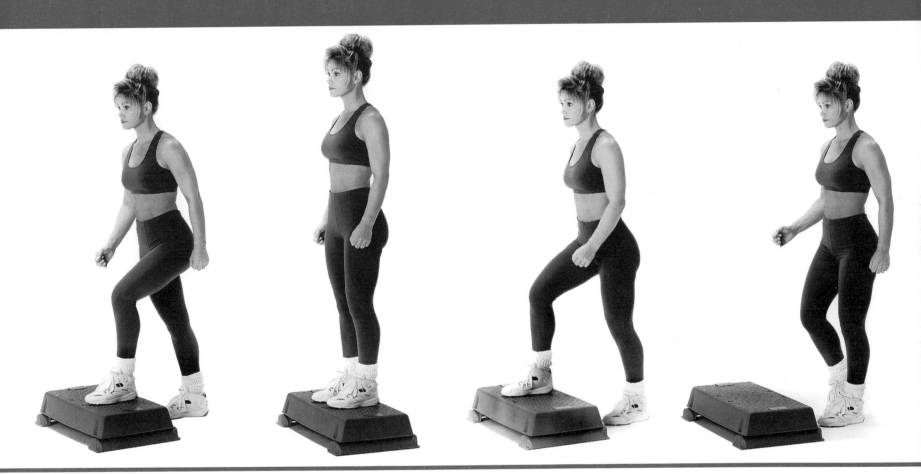

5 Return your LEFT foot to the platform, ball to heel. Make sure your foot position is square and solid.

6 Step up with your RIGHT foot. Your weight should be evenly distributed between both feet over the center of the platform.

7 Lift your LEFT foot and step down to the floor behind the center of the platform, ball to heel.

8 Lift your RIGHT foot from the platform and TAP DOWN with your RIGHT toe on the floor about 6 inches from your left foot. You are now in a position to repeat the pattern or go on to another one.

ALTERNATING TAP UP

This pattern is similar to the Alternating Tap Down, but instead of alternately tapping down on the floor, you tap up on the platform to change lead-off legs.

Step Stats

- 8 beats
- Starting position: Front
- Repetitions: 4 (32 beats)

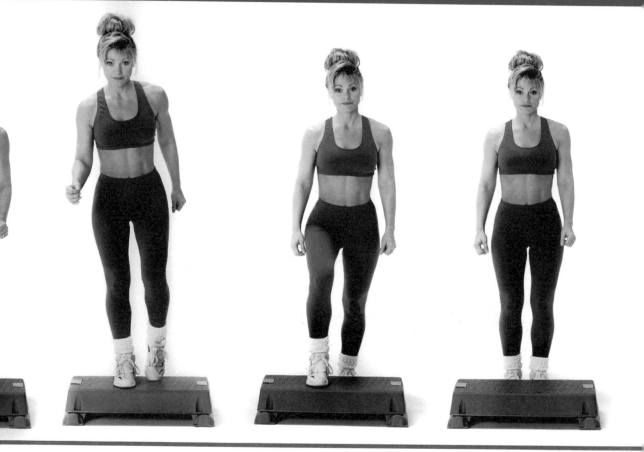

1 From the front starting position, lift your RIGHT foot and step squarely on the middle of the platform, ball to heel.

2 Lift your LEFT foot and TAP UP with your LEFT toe near the center of the platform about 6 inches away from your right foot. Don't step up, just tap. Be careful not to lock your knees.

3 Return your LEFT foot to its starting position on the floor behind the middle of the platform.

4 Lift your RIGHT foot from the platform and return it to its starting position on the floor, ball to heel. Both feet are on the floor now, about 6 inches apart.

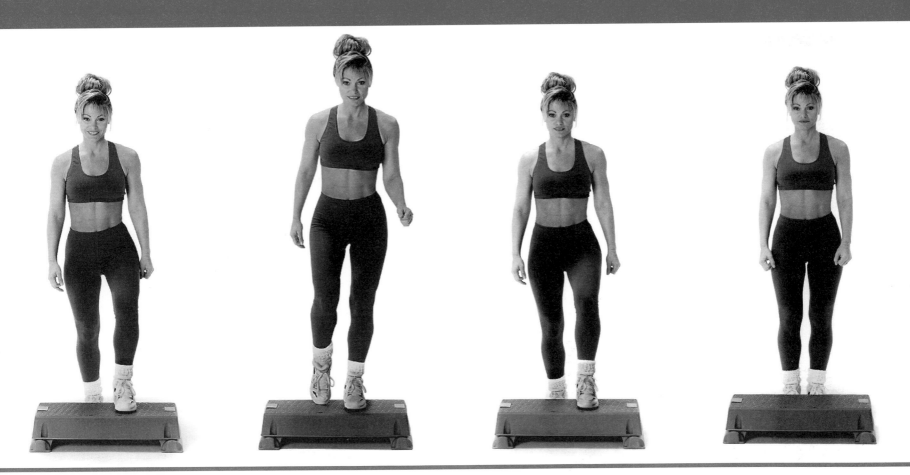

5 Lift your LEFT foot and step up squarely on the middle of the platform, ball to heel.

6 Lift your RIGHT foot and TAP UP with your RIGHT toe on the center of the platform about 6 inches away from your left foot. Don't step up, just tap.

7 Return your RIGHT foot to the floor behind the center of the platform. Be careful not to lock your knees.

8 Return your LEFT foot to the floor, ball to heel. Stand with your weight equally distributed between both feet.

ALTERNATING WIDE-STEP TAP DOWN

This pattern combines the Wide Step with the Alternating Tap Down. You lead off with both legs alternately tapping down on the floor and stepping wide on the platform.

Step Stats

- 8 beats
- Starting position: Front
- Repetitions: 4 (32 beats)

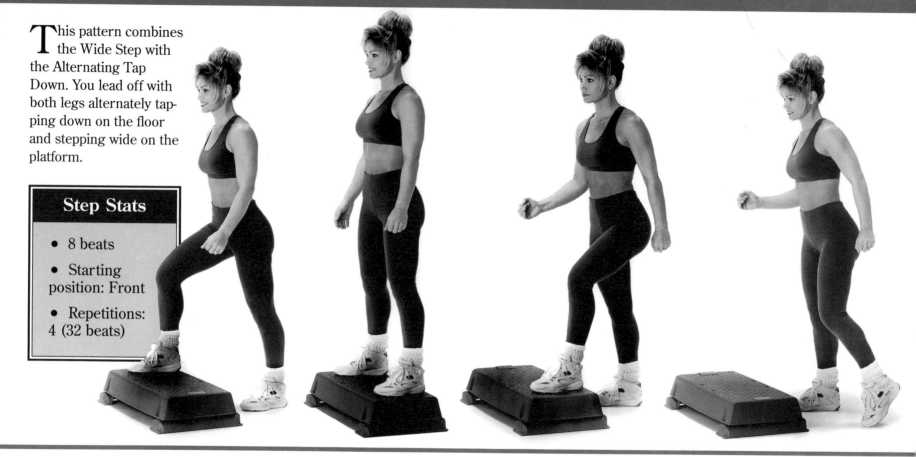

1 From the front starting position, lift your RIGHT foot and step squarely on the RIGHT end of the platform, ball to heel. Keep your fists loose and let your arms swing naturally.

2 Step up with your LEFT foot on the LEFT end of the platform, ball to heel. You should be standing with your feet wide apart on top of the platform, your weight equally distributed between them.

3 Return your RIGHT foot to the floor behind the center of the platform.

4 Lift your LEFT foot from the platform and TAP DOWN on the floor with your LEFT toe.

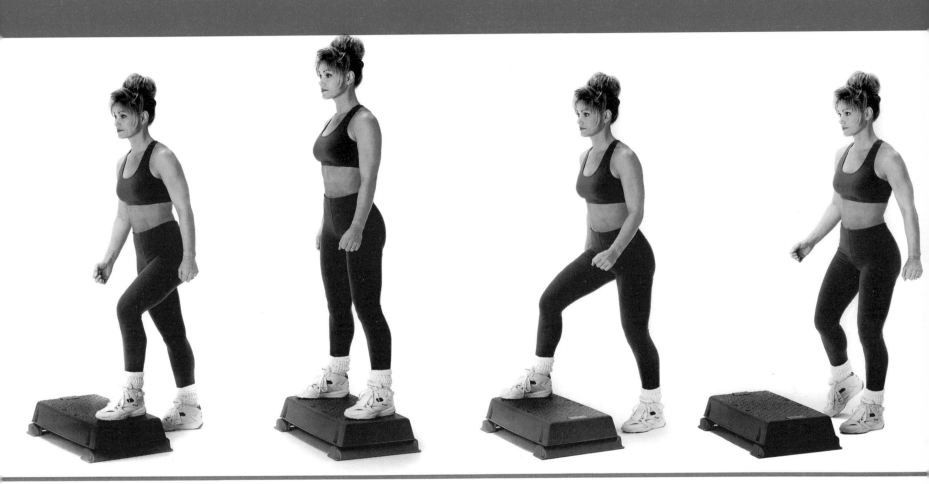

5 Return your LEFT foot to the LEFT end of the platform.

6 Return your RIGHT foot to the RIGHT end of the platform. You should be standing with both feet flat and wide apart on the top of the platform with your weight equally distributed.

7 Lift your LEFT foot from the platform and return it to the floor behind the center of the platform, ball to heel.

8 Lift your RIGHT foot from the platform and TAP DOWN on the floor with your RIGHT toe next to your left foot. Now you are in position to repeat the pattern or start a new one.

ALTERNATING KNEE LIFT

This is the first step pattern where you lift your leg away from the platform while you are on top. The movement of lifting the knee exercises and strengthens the hip flexors. Both legs will lead off in this pattern.

Step Stats

- 8 beats
- Starting position: Front
- Repetitions: 4 (32 beats)

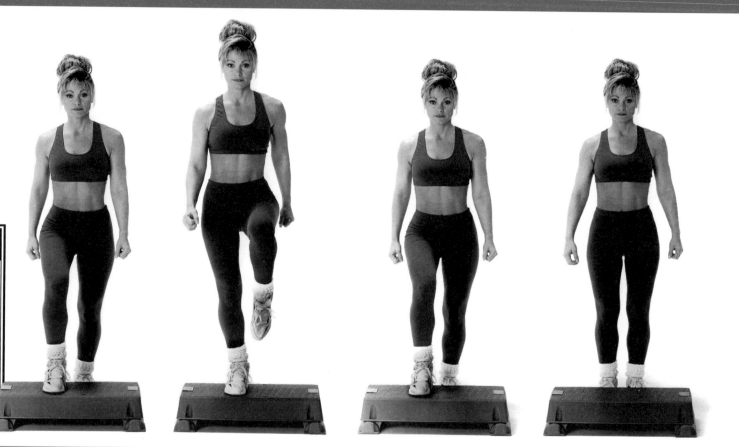

1 From the front starting position, lift your RIGHT foot and step squarely on the middle of the platform, ball to heel.

2 Lift your LEFT foot until your LEFT knee forms a 90° angle.

3 Lower your LEFT foot to its starting position on the floor, ball to heel.

4 Lift your RIGHT foot from the platform and return it to the floor, ball to heel. Your feet should be about 6 inches apart. Keep your back straight and your chin up.

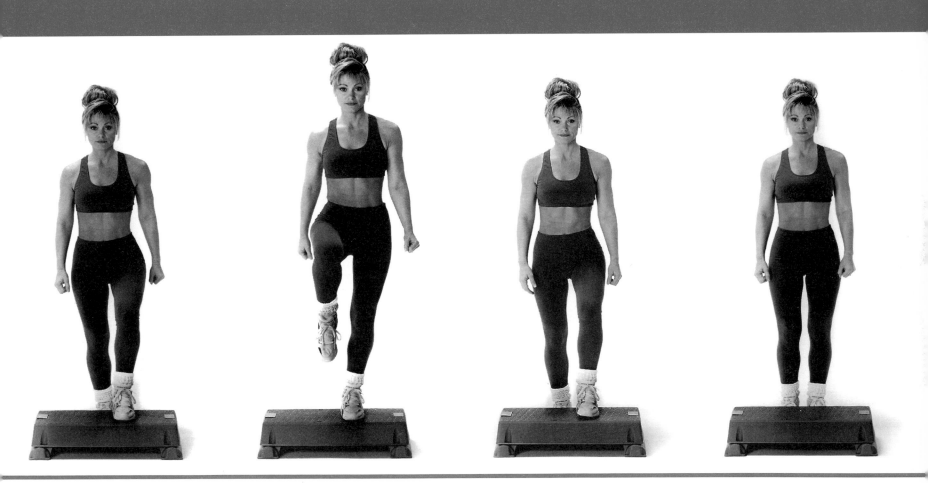

5 Lift your LEFT foot and step squarely on the center of the platform, ball to heel.

6 Lift your RIGHT foot until your RIGHT knee forms a 90° angle.

7 Lower your RIGHT foot to its starting position on the floor, ball to heel.

8 Lift your LEFT foot from the platform and return it to the floor, ball to heel. Stand in the starting position with your weight equally distributed between both feet.

ALTERNATING LEG LIFT

This pattern is similar to the alternating knee lift but by lifting the whole leg to the side, you are working the muscles of the outer thigh. Both legs will lead off in this pattern.

Step Stats

- 8 beats
- Starting position: Front
- Repetitions: 4 (32 beats)

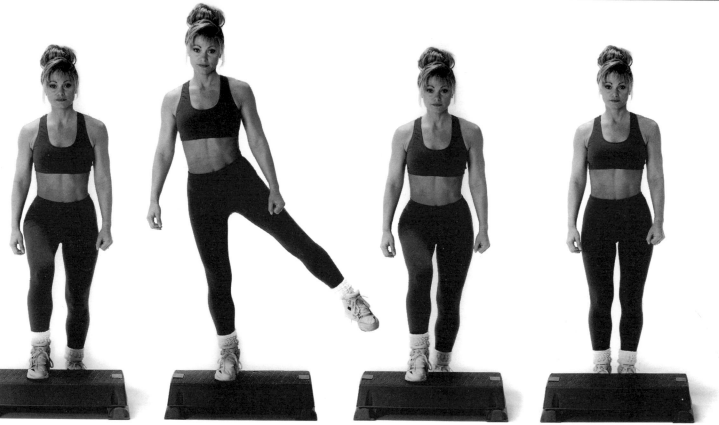

1 From the front starting position, lift your RIGHT foot and step squarely on the center of the platform, ball to heel.

2 Lift your LEFT leg straight out to the side, keeping your knee straight but not locked. Don't let your body lean to the side.

3 Return your LEFT foot to the floor in the same position as the starting position.

4 Lift your RIGHT foot from the platform and return it to the floor, ball to heel, so you're standing in the starting position, with your weight equally distributed.

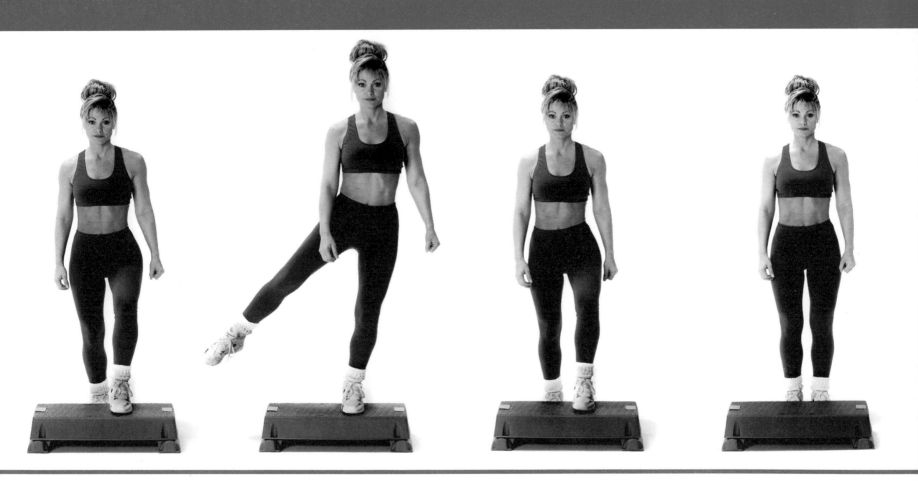

5 Lift your LEFT foot and step squarely on the center of the platform, ball to heel.

6 Lift your RIGHT leg straight out to the side, keeping your knee straight but not locked. Don't let your body lean to the side.

7 Return your RIGHT foot to the floor in the same position as the starting position.

8 Lift your LEFT foot from the platform and return it to the floor, ball to heel. Stand in the starting position ready to repeat the pattern or start a new one.

ALTERNATING HEEL LIFT

As in the Alternating Knee Lift and the Alternating Leg Lift, you alternate leading legs. But in this pattern, you lift your heels behind you to work the hamstring muscles in the back of the thigh.

Step Stats

- 8 beats
- Starting position: Front
- Repetitions: 4 (32 beats)

1 From the front starting position, lift your RIGHT foot and step squarely on the center of the platform, ball to heel.

2 Lift your LEFT heel up behind you. The line from your hip to your knee should be straight down.

3 Return your LEFT foot to the floor behind the center of the platform.

4 Return your RIGHT foot to the floor so that you're standing in the starting position with your weight equally distributed.

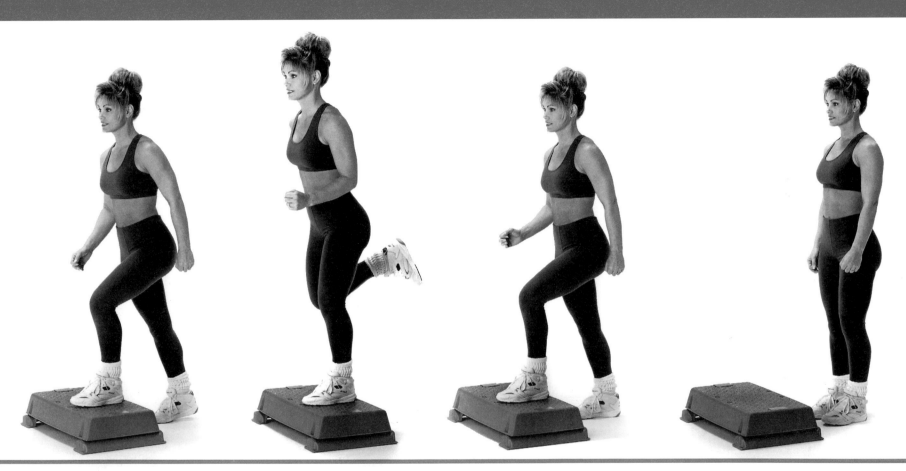

5 Step up with your LEFT foot to the center of the platform, ball to heel.

6 Lift your RIGHT heel up behind you. Remember, the line from your hip to your knee should be straight down.

7 Return your RIGHT foot to the floor behind the center of the platform.

8 Lift your LEFT foot and return it to the floor, ball to heel. You should be in the front starting position with your weight distributed between both feet.

TURN

This pattern is a "traveling" Alternating Wide-Step Tap Down. You face one direction, move to face the other direction and then return. The turn works all the muscles of the leg.

Step Stats

- 8 beats
- Starting position: Side
- Repetitions: 4 (beats)

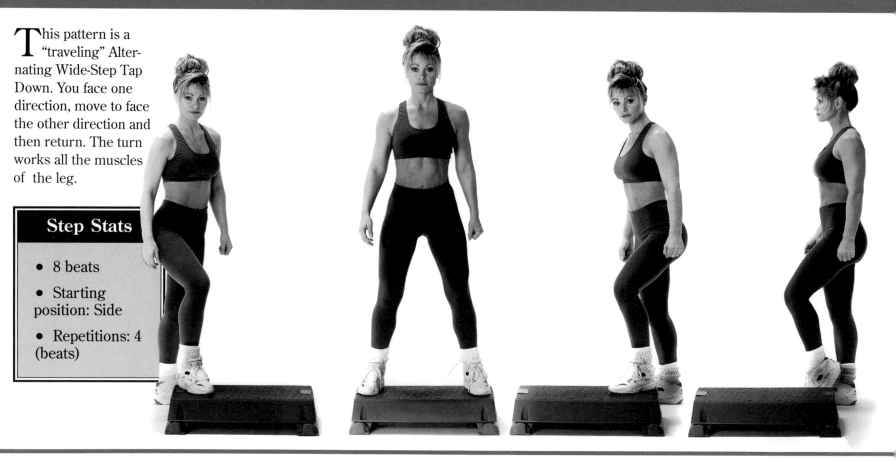

1 From the side starting position with the long edge of the platform to your right, lift your RIGHT foot and step squarely on the RIGHT end of the platform, ball to heel. Your toes should be pointed toward the front.

2 Lift your LEFT foot, turn your body until you are facing front, and step up on the LEFT end of the platform, ball to heel. Stand with both feet flat on the platform, body facing forward, weight equally distributed.

3 Lift your RIGHT foot from the platform and turn your body while you return your foot to the floor on the LEFT side of the platform. Your body should now be in the position opposite to the one you started in.

4 Lift your LEFT foot and TAP DOWN on the floor. The long edge of the platform should now be to your left.

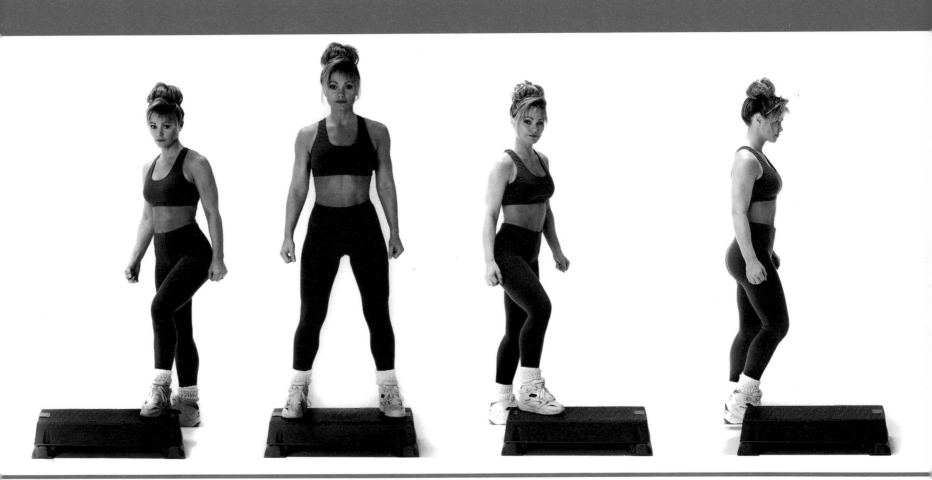

5 With the platform to your left, lift your LEFT foot and step up on the LEFT end of the platform. Your toes should be pointing to the front, and you should begin to turn your body to the front.

6 Lift your RIGHT foot, turn your body until your are facing the front, and step up on the RIGHT end of the platform, ball to heel. Stand with both feet flat on the platform, body facing front.

7 Lift your LEFT foot from the platform and turn your body to the left while you return your foot to the floor as it was in the original starting position.

8 Lift your RIGHT foot and TAP DOWN with your RIGHT TOE on the floor. You are now in a position to repeat the pattern or go on to another one.

OVER THE TOP

This is a simple step pattern that gets you over the top of the platform. It works the quadriceps, calves, and hamstrings as it takes you from one side of the platform to the other.

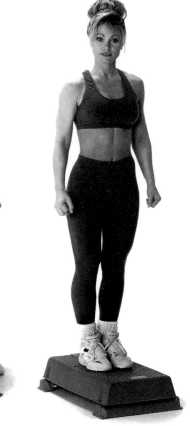
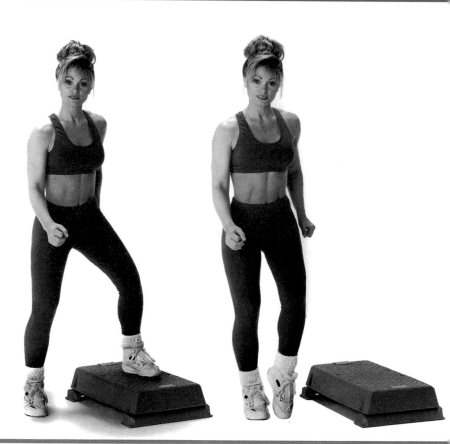

Step Stats

- 8 beats
- Starting position: Side
- Repetitions: 4 (32 beats)

1 From the side starting position with the long edge of the platform to your right, lift your RIGHT foot and step up on the center of the platform, ball to heel with your toes pointed to the short edge of the platform.

2 Lift your LEFT foot and step up, ball to heel, so that you're standing sideways on the platform with BOTH feet flat and your weight equally distributed between them.

3 Lift your RIGHT foot and step down to the floor on the side of the platform opposite to the one you started from. Let your arms swing naturally.

4 Lift your LEFT foot from the platform and TAP DOWN on the floor with your LEFT toe between your right foot and the platform.

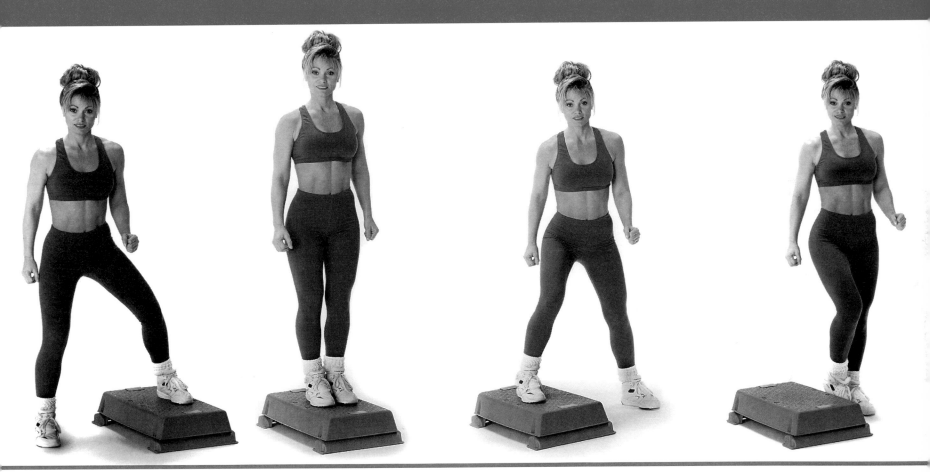

5 Return your LEFT foot to the platform, ball to heel.

6 Lift your RIGHT foot and step up on the platform.

7 Lift your LEFT foot from the platform and return it to the floor on the starting position side of platform.

8 Lift your RIGHT foot from the platform and TAP DOWN on the floor with your RIGHT toe between your left foot and the platform. This puts you into a position to repeat this pattern or begin another.

TAP UP/TAP DOWN

This is a basic four-beat pattern where you tap up on the platform and tap down on the floor. This pattern works both the gluteus medius and adductor muscles of the outer and the inner thigh.

Step Stats

- 4 beats
- Starting position: Front
- Repetitions: 8 (32 beats)

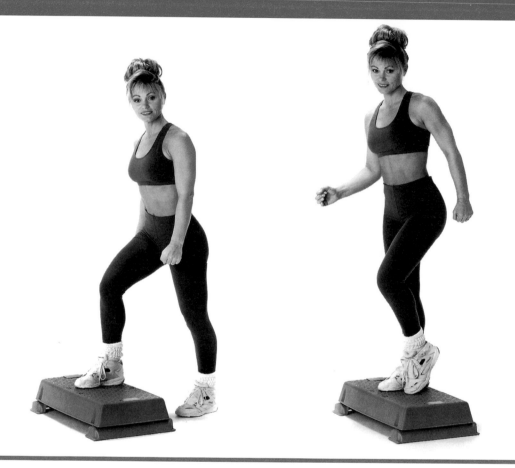

1 From the front starting position, lift your RIGHT foot and step up squarely on the center of the platform, ball to heel.

2 Lift your LEFT foot and TAP UP on the platform with your LEFT toe. Keep your chin up, and let your arms swing naturally.

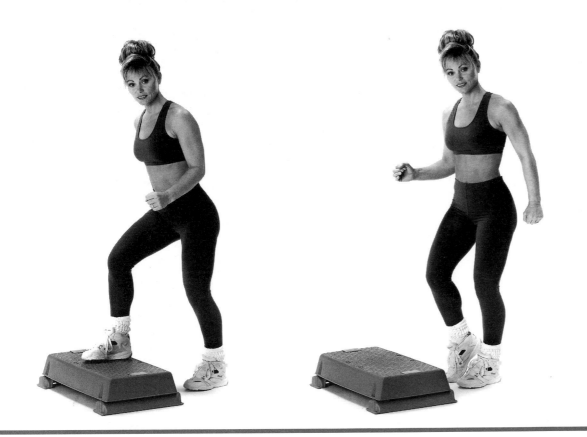

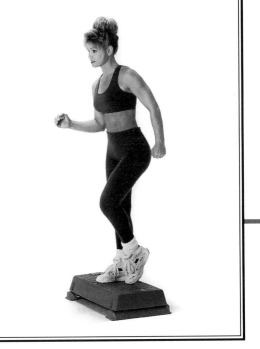

PROPER TAP TECHNIQUE

Your weight is always centered when you tap up or down. Never put your full weight on the tapping foot. The heel of the tapping foot doesn't come in contact with the floor because the resulting stretch would cause a shift in weight and might strain ligaments and tendons in the foot and heel.

3 Return your LEFT foot to the floor behind the center of the platform.

4 TAP DOWN on the floor with your RIGHT toe. Now you are in a position to repeat this pattern or begin another.

REPEATER

Lifting the same leg three times in a row is called a repeater. A repeater can be used with a Tap, Leg Lift, Knee Lift, or Heel Lift. The example here is a Repeater Knee Lift. This pattern is a strengthening move for the quadriceps, hamstrings and buttocks.

Step Stats

- 8 beats
- Starting position: Front
- Repetitions: 4 (32 beats)

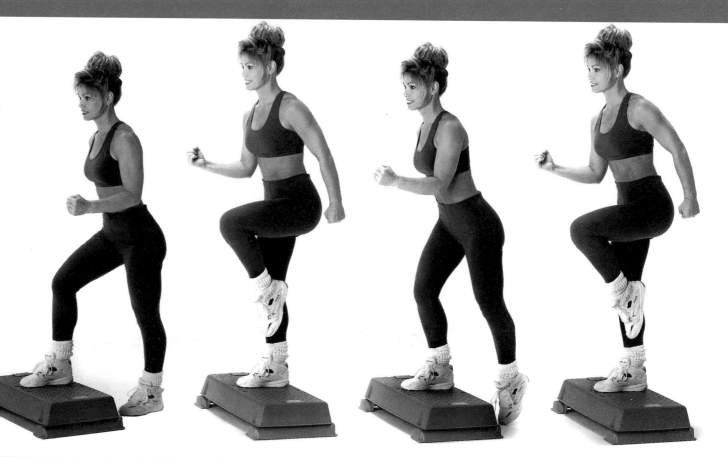

1 From the front starting position, lift your RIGHT foot and step up squarely on the center of the platform, ball to heel. Your weight remains on the same foot throughout this pattern.

2 Lift your LEFT foot until your LEFT knee forms a 90° angle. Your arms will swing naturally.

3 Bring your LEFT foot back to the floor and TAP DOWN with your LEFT toe.

4 Lift your LEFT knee.

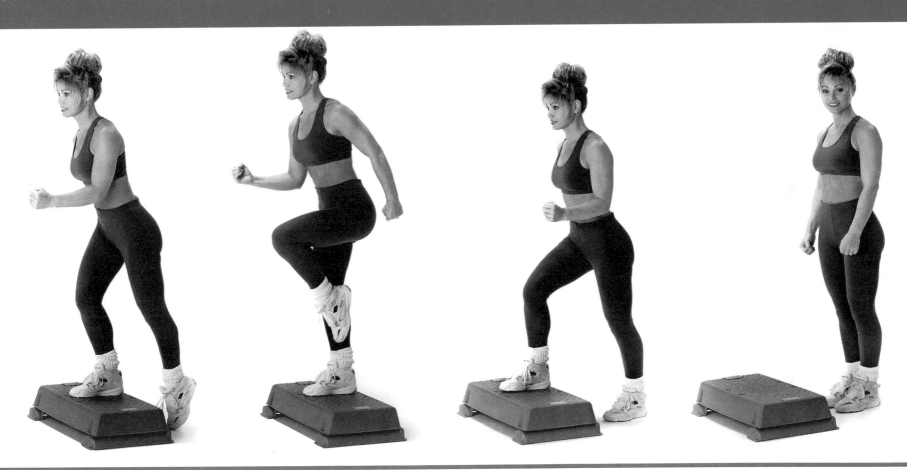

5 TAP DOWN with your LEFT toe.

6 Lift your LEFT knee.

7 After lifting three times, step down with your LEFT foot on the floor directly behind the platform.

8 Step down with your RIGHT foot on the floor directly behind the platform. You should be back in the starting position, ready to repeat this pattern with your RIGHT leg.

ALTERNATING LUNGE

In this pattern, you begin by standing on top of the platform. By alternately lunging and extending each leg behind you off the platform, you bring your heart rate up and work the quadriceps and calves. When extending the lunging leg, barely touch your toes on the floor.

Step Stats

- 4 beats
- Starting position: Top
- Repetitions: 8 (32 beats)

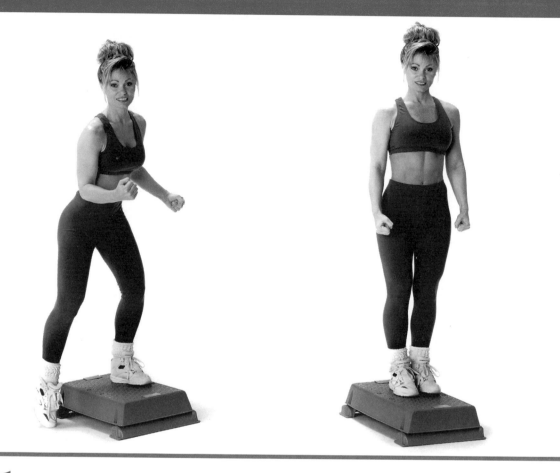

1 From the top starting position, lift your RIGHT foot from the platform and TAP DOWN on the right side of the platform. Keep your back straight and your shoulders square.

2 Return your RIGHT foot to the top starting position.

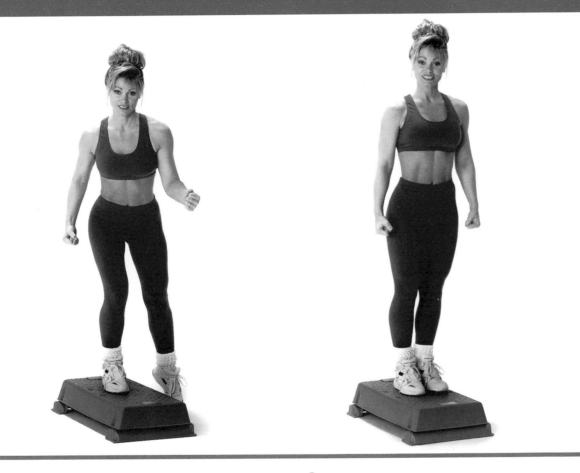

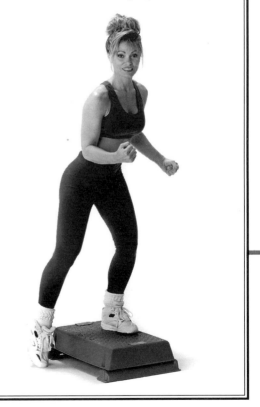

PROTECT YOUR JOINTS

When you lunge, keep your weight forward over your supporting leg. Keeping both knees slightly bent and your weight forward protects not only your knees and ankles, it also prevents lower back injury.

3 Lift your LEFT foot from the platform and TAP DOWN on the LEFT side of the platform. Again, keep your back straight and your shoulders squared.

4 Return your LEFT foot to the top starting position.

STRADDLE DOWN

This pattern begins on top of the platform. The movement is similar to the Basic Right and Wide Step, but you step down on either side of the platform in a straddle position while you work both the inner and outer thigh.

Step Stats

- 4 beats
- Starting position: Top
- Repetitions: 8 (32 beats)

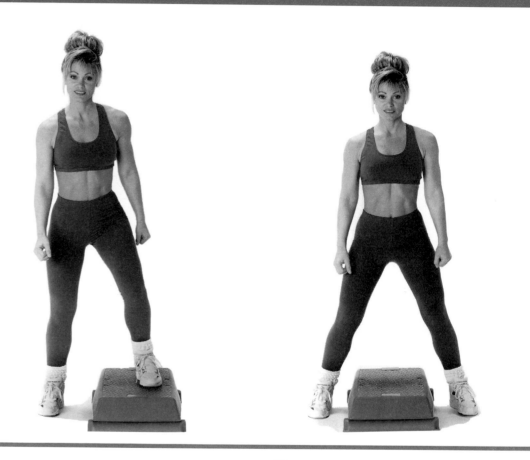

1 From the top starting position, lift your RIGHT foot and step down to the floor on the right side of the platform.

2 Lift your LEFT foot and step down to the floor on the LEFT side of the platform.

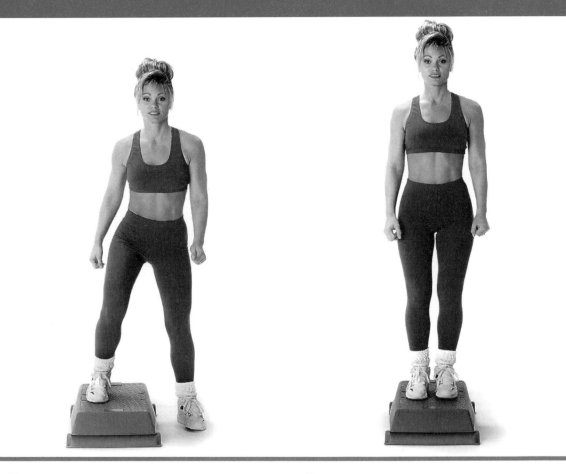

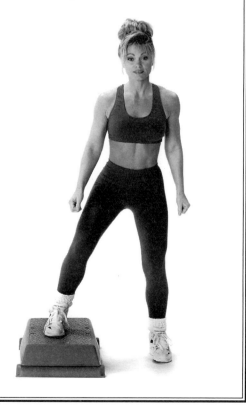

3 Lift your RIGHT foot from the floor and step squarely on the top of the platform, ball to heel.

4 Lift your LEFT foot from the floor and step squarely on the top of the platform, ball to heel. Stand with your weight equally distributed between both feet.

THE FIRST STEP

When you straddle the platform, don't step too far away with the leading leg or you might pull a muscle by stretching too far with the other leg. Always step down about 6 inches away from the edge, and keep your body centered over the center of the platform.

ALTERNATING TAP UP/STRADDLE DOWN

This pattern is a combination of the Straddle Down and the Alternating Tap. You begin on the top of the step and straddle down, but you alternate legs and tap instead of step. This pattern can be done with added Knee, Leg, and Heel Lifts.

Step Stats

- 8 beats
- Starting position: Top
- Repetitions: 8 (32 beats)

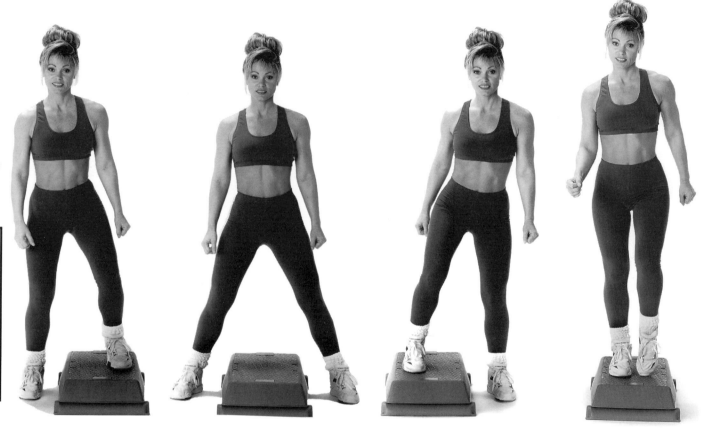

1 From the top starting position, lift your RIGHT foot and step down to the floor on the right side of the platform, ball to heel.

2 Lift your LEFT foot and step down to the floor on the left side of the platform, ball to heel, so that you are straddling the platform with your weight equally distributed on both feet.

3 Lift your RIGHT foot and return it to the starting position on the top of the platform.

4 Lift your LEFT foot and TAP UP on the platform with your LEFT toe. Don't step, just tap.

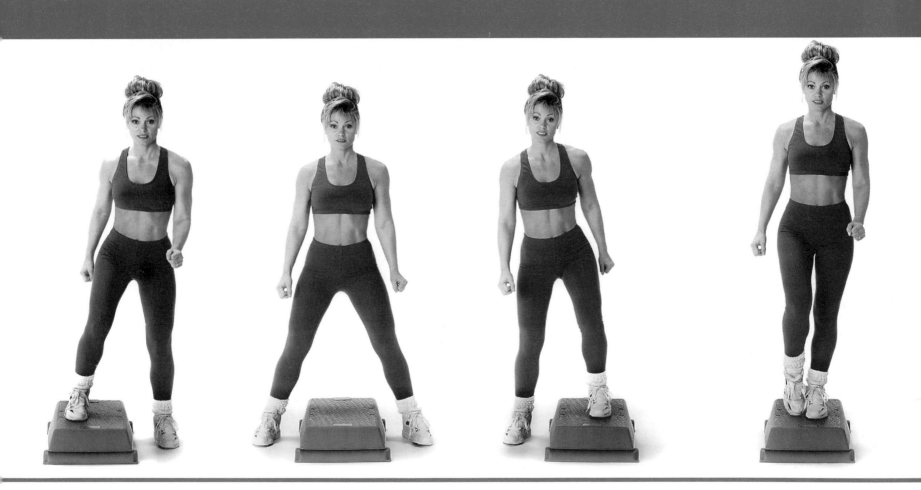

5 Step down with your LEFT foot on the left side of the platform.

6 Step down with your RIGHT foot on the floor to the right of the platform.

7 Lift your LEFT foot and step up on the platform.

8 Lift your RIGHT foot and TAP UP. You will be in a position to repeat the pattern or begin a new one.

ACROSS THE TOP

This pattern is the same as Over the Top, except that you start at one end of the platform and move across it the long way.

Step Stats

- 8 beats
- Starting position: End
- Repetitions: 4 (32 beats)

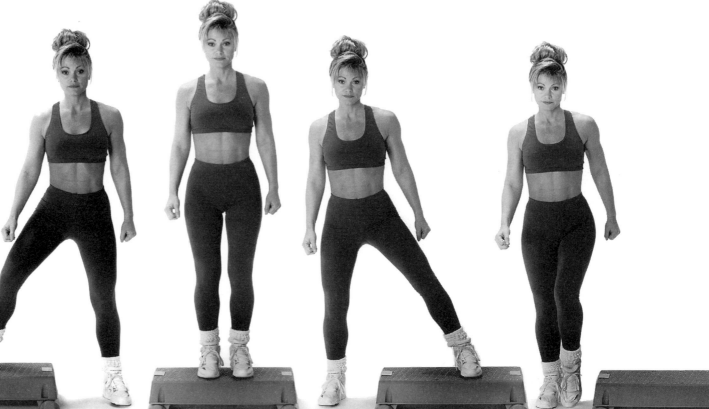

1 From the end starting position with the platform to your right, lift your RIGHT foot and step up on the center of the platform, ball to heel.

2 Step up on the platform with your LEFT foot, ball to heel, so that you're standing with both feet in the center of the platform, your weight equally distributed on both legs.

3 Lift your RIGHT foot and step down on the floor to the right of the platform. Step far enough over so that your left foot can tap down between your right foot and the platform.

4 Lift your LEFT foot and TAP DOWN between your right foot and the platform.

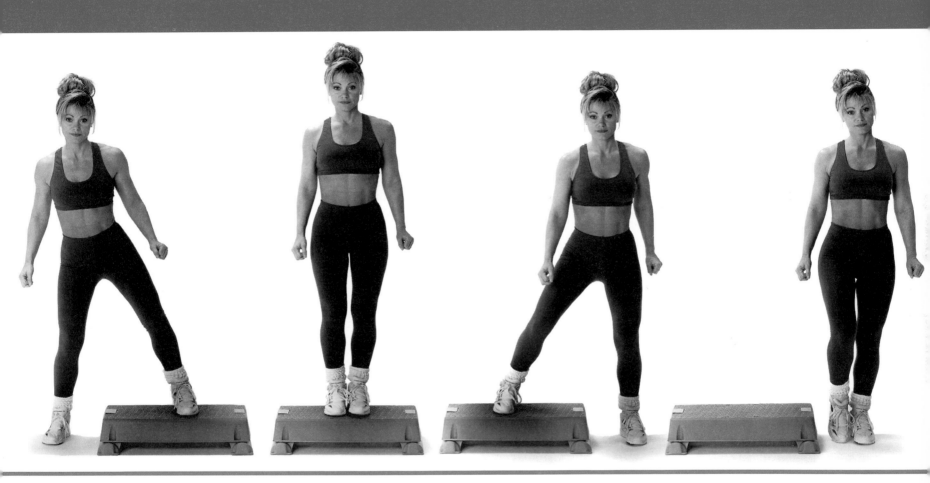

5 Lift your LEFT foot and step back up on the center of the platform.

6 Lift your RIGHT foot and step up on the platform.

7 Lift your LEFT foot and step down.

8 Lift your RIGHT foot from the platform and TAP DOWN. You should be in the starting position, ready to repeat the pattern or begin a new one.

"A little extra effort makes a lot of difference."

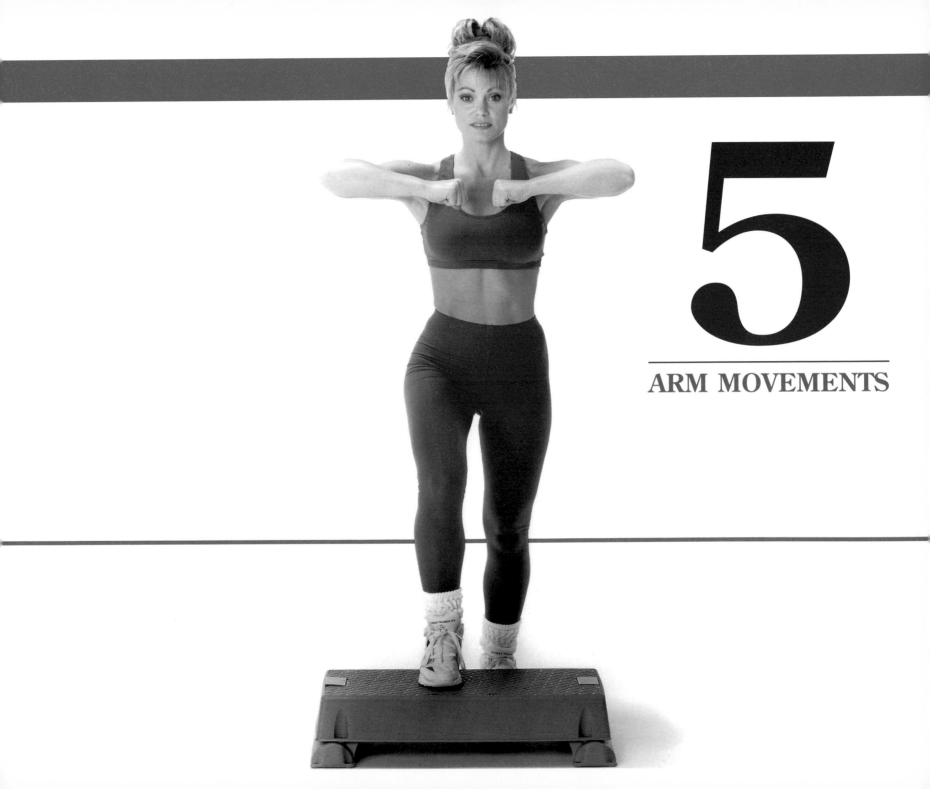

5

ARM MOVEMENTS

CHAPTER 5

ARM MOVEMENTS

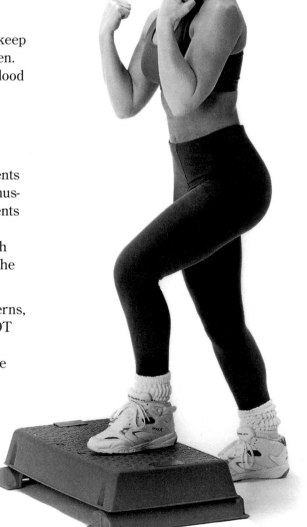

Arm movements
raise your heart rate
and benefit arm,
shoulder and upper
back muscles.

When you have gained confidence in the step patterns, you may want to add arm movements to increase the intensity of your aerobic workout.

Unless you work out with weights strenuously and frequently, your arms get neglected in exercise. Your upper arms (the biceps and the triceps) are the first thing to sag, no matter how fit you may be, unless you work them frequently. The shoulder and upper back muscle groups are also often ignored, resulting in stiffness and stooping. Good posture and an upright stance depend on having strong, healthy muscles of the shoulders and upper back.

One way to help firm up the flabbiness and relieve tension is to add powerful arm movements to your workout. And the best way to strengthen the muscles of the upper torso is by performing body-sculpting exercises (Chapter 6) using resistance in the form of weights or rubber bands.

Adding arm movements to your workout accomplishes two things. By exercising the muscle groups of your upper body, you deplete the oxygen supply faster and increase your heart rate as it strives to keep up with the increased demand for oxygen. When your heart rate increases, your blood is pumped at a faster rate and your breathing rate also increases. Overall, including arm movements significantly elevates the intensity of your workout.

The other advantage of arm movements is the benefit to the arm and shoulder muscles themselves. Although arm movements don't in any way replace body sculpting (Chapter 6), performing them along with the step patterns does help strengthen the upper body.

Once you have learned the step patterns, it's easy to add arm movements. DO NOT add arm movements until you have mastered the step patterns. If at any time

"Adding arm movements increases the intensity of your workout."

you feel dizzy or overwhelmed, go back to stepping without arm movements until you build up strength and endurance.

Often constant repetitiveness can cause discomfort. Never use hand weights during the aerobic or cardiovascular part of your workout. The extra weights can do damage to joints and tendons. There are far more benefits to using the hand weights in the body-sculpting exercises. You can, however, boost the benefits of the arm movements used with step patterns by moving your arms with strength and power.

The arm movements on the following pages work the muscles of the upper body. They are presented in terms of moving both arms at once or alternating arm movements. The basic movements are all shown with the Basic Right step pattern. Each arm movement can be repeated in sequence for any of the described step patterns in Chapter 4. Repeat the arm movements in sequence for however many pairs of beats in the accompanying step pattern.

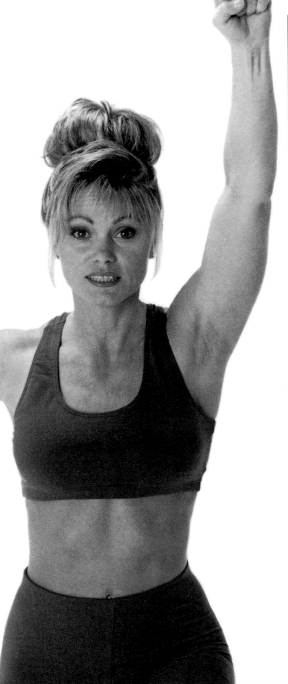

Arm movements as well as body sculpting exercises strengthen the upper body.

Safety Tips

- To avoid stress on the shoulder girdle, don't maintain the arms at or above the shoulder level for an extended period of time.

- Never lock your elbows or overextend them. Over stretching could cause pain and injury.

- Make fists, but don't clench.

- The arm movements should be smooth and continuous. Don't throw your arms into position. Keep them strong and in control.

- If you feel dizzy or overwhelmed, stop arm movements.

- Stop arm movements if you feel pain.

BICEPS CURL

The Biceps Curl is the simplest arm movement and the least intensive. It puts no stress on the shoulder or upper back as the movements are made below shoulder level.

Arm Stats

• Use the Biceps Curl with the Basic Right or Basic Left, Alternating Knee Lift, and Tap Up/Tap Down.

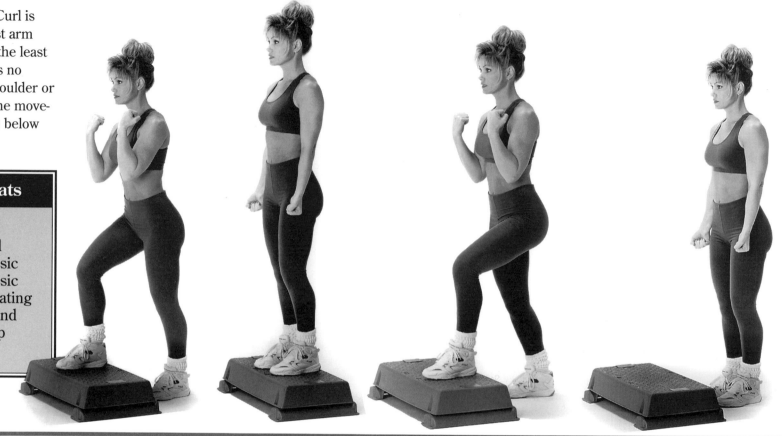

1 Starting with your arms straight down, hands in a fist, curl both arms toward your shoulders. Your fists face your body.

2 Straighten both arms down so they are next to your body. Your fists face up.

3 Curl both arms toward your shoulders again.

4 Straighten both arms.

ALTERNATING BICEPS CURL

The Alternating Biceps Curl is essentially the same as the Biceps Curl except that you alternate arms.

Arm Stats

• Use the Alternating Biceps Curl with the Basic Right or Basic Left, Alternating Knee Lift, and Tap Up/Tap Down.

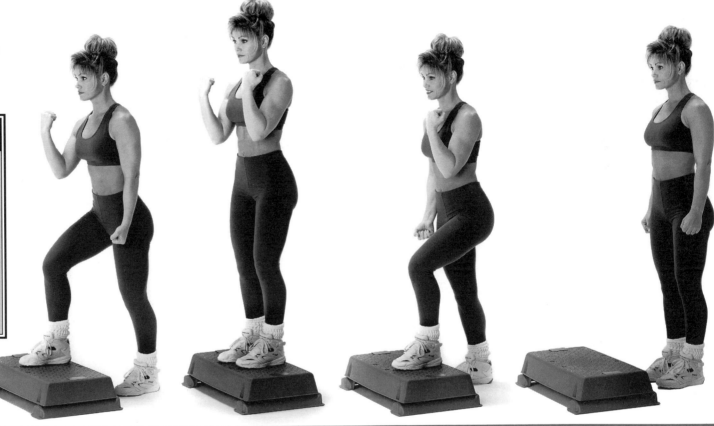

1 Starting with your arms straight down, hands in a fist and facing upward, curl your right forearm toward your shoulder. Leave the left arm straight.

2 Curl your left arm toward your shoulder. Both arms are now curled.

3 Return your right arm to your side.

4 Return your left arm to your side.

SHOULDER PUNCH

The Shoulder Punch works the muscles of the upper arm and shoulder and intensifies your workout.

Arm Stats

• Use the Shoulder Punch with Alternating Knee Lift, Straddle Down, Tap Up/Tap Down, Over the Top, and Alternating Lunge.

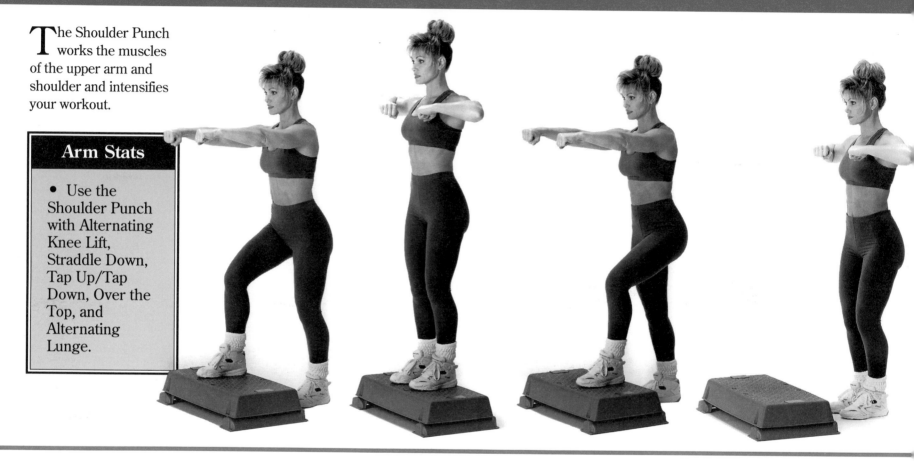

1 Extend both arms outward in front of you until they are straight, with hands in a fist. Make sure the elbows are not locked. Your pelvis should be tucked under and your chin lifted.

2 Keeping your elbows out and your arms parallel to the floor, bring both fists back toward your chest.

3 Extend the arms again, making sure not to lock the elbows.

4 Return both arms to the bent position.

ALTERNATING SHOULDER PUNCH

The Alternating Shoulder Punch is essentially the same as the Shoulder Punch except that you alternate arms. Lead off with the right arm for both punching and withdrawing.

Arm Stats

• Use the Alternating Shoulder Punch with Alternating Knee Lift, Straddle Down, Tap Up/Tap Down, Over the Top, and Alternating Lunge.

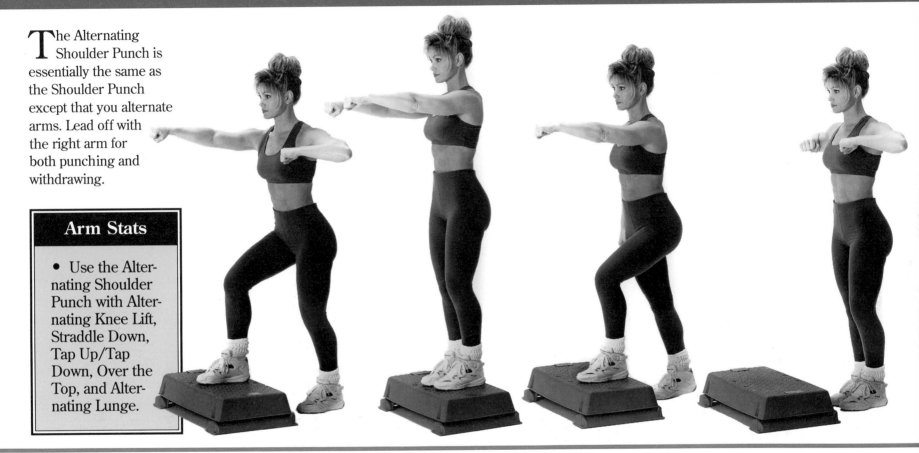

1 Punch forward with your right arm while leaving your left arm in the bent position.

2 Punch forward with your left arm so that both arms are extended.

3 Bring back your right arm to the bent position.

4 Bring back your left arm to the bent position.

OVERHEAD PRESS

The Overhead Press works the muscles in the shoulder and upper arm. It is the most strenuous of the arm movements, as the motion is above shoulder level.

Arm Stats

• Use the Overhead Press with the Alternating Knee Lift, Straddle Down, Across the Top, Over the Top, Alternating Leg Lift and Alternating Lunge.

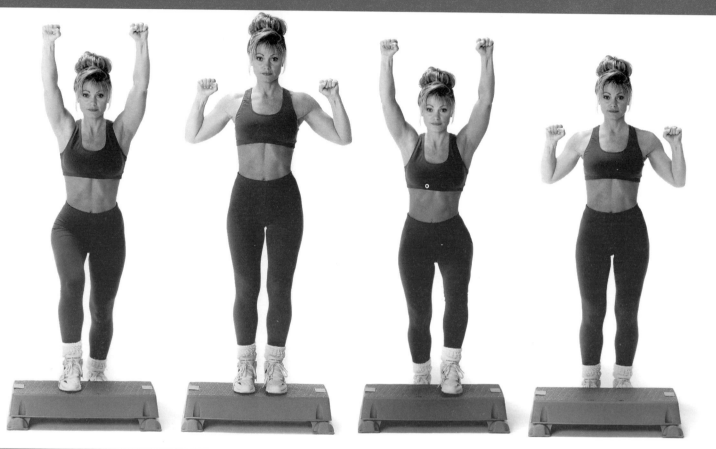

1 Extend both arms straight up over your head, hands in a fist. Keep your fists facing forward and don't lock your elbows.

2 Bend your arms until your fists are at shoulder level. Your fists should face forward during the entire movement.

3 Extend your arms up again.

4 Return both arms to the bent position.

ALTERNATING OVERHEAD PRESS

The Alternating Overhead Press works the same muscle groups as the Overhead Press as you alternate arms.

Arm Stats

• Use the Alternating Overhead Press with the Alternating Knee Lift, Straddle Down, Across the Top, Over the Top, Alternating Leg Lift and Alternating Lunge.

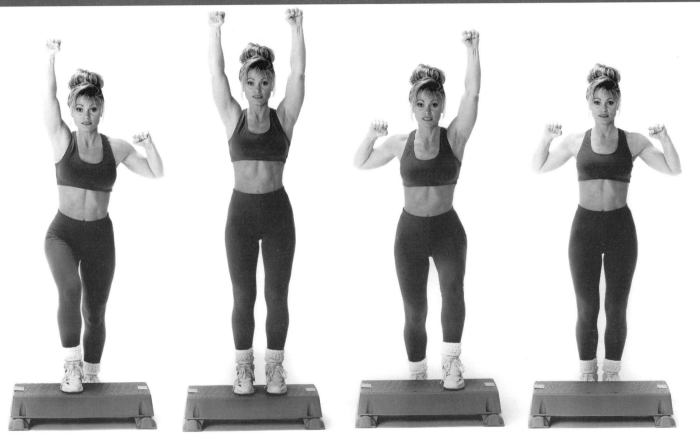

1 With hands in a fist, extend your right arm over your head, keeping your left arm bent. Both fists face forward.

2 Extend your left arm overhead so that both arms are straight up and fists face forward.

3 Bend your right arm so that the elbow is straight out and the fist is shoulder level.

4 Bend your left arm so that both fists are shoulder level.

UPRIGHT ROW

The Upright Row exercises the major muscles of the upper arms and back. In this movement, imagine you are pulling up on a rope. Your elbows come up first as you draw both arms up to chest level.

Arm Stats

- Use the Upright Row with the Turn, Wide Step, Basic Right, and Basic Left.

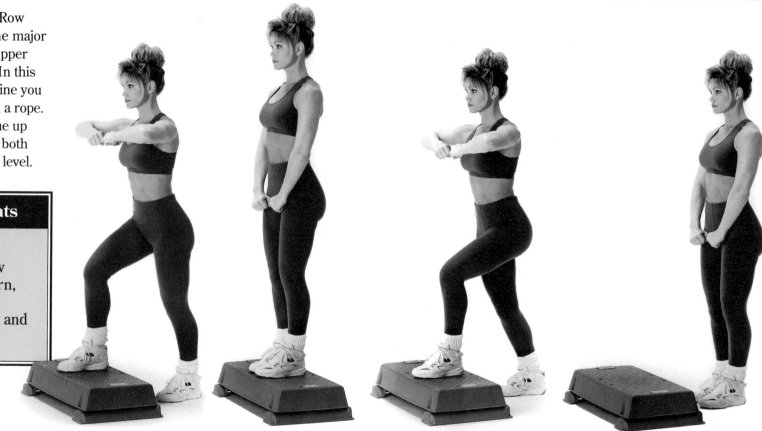

1 Starting with both arms straight, hands in a fist, pull arms up to shoulder level, keeping your fists close to your body and your elbows out to the side.

2 Extend both arms down the sides of your body. Your fists should face down and your elbows should be slightly bent.

3 Pull both arms up again, keeping your fists facing down.

4 Return both arms to the straight position.

ALTERNATING UPRIGHT ROW

The Alternating Upright Row works the same muscle groups as the Upright Row as you alternate arms. Lead with your right arm in both raising and lowering.

Arm Stats

- Use the Alternating Upright Row with the Turn, Wide Step, Basic Right and Basic Left.

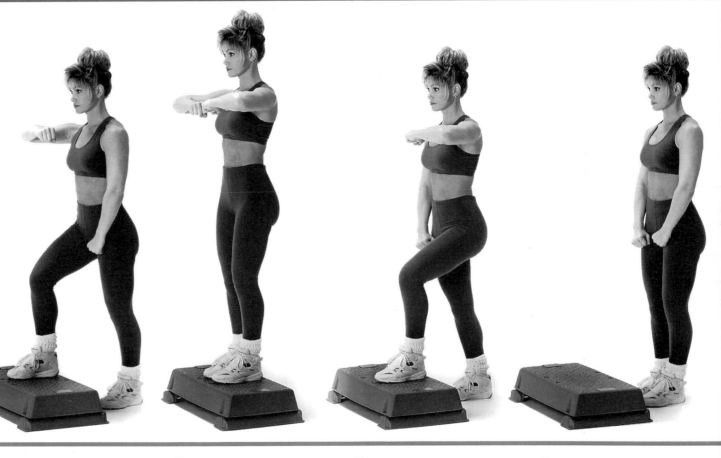

1 Starting with both arms down, hands in a fist, pull your right arm up to shoulder level, elbow out to your side, fist close to your shoulder.

2 Pull your left arm up to mirror your right arm.

3 Return your right arm to your side.

4 Return your left arm to your side.

TRICEPS KICK BACK

The Triceps Kick Back is the only arm movement performed behind your back. It exercises the triceps muscles in the upper arm.

Arm Stats

- Use the Triceps Kick Back with the Alternating Heel Lift and Tap Up/Tap Down patterns.

1 Extend your arms straight out behind you, hands in a fist. Your elbows should point up and your fists should face into your body.

2 Bend both arms until your fists are next to your ribs and your elbows are bent and pointing straight back.

3 Extend your arms back again making sure your elbows don't lock.

4 Return both arms to the bent position.

ALTERNATING TRICEPS KICK BACK

The Alternating Triceps Kick Back works the same muscle groups as the Triceps Kick Back as you alternate arms. Lead with your right arm when you extend and when you bend your arms.

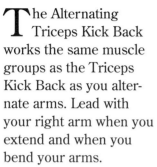
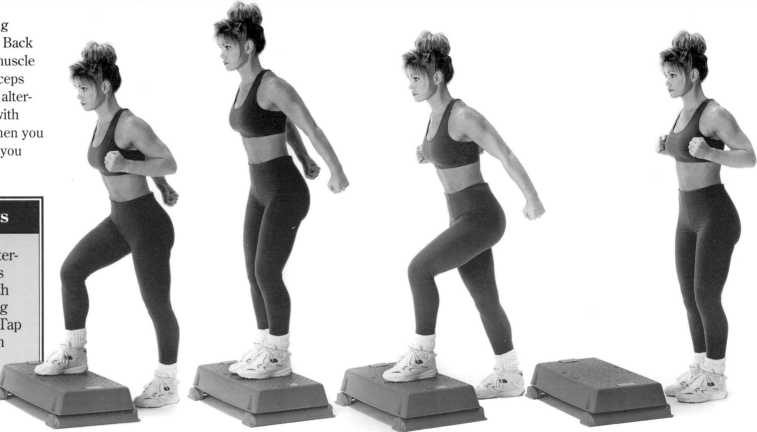

1 Starting with both arms bent close to your body, hands in a fist, extend your right arm back and up. Keep your left arm bent and close to your side.

2 Extend your left arm back and up so that both arms are straight back, fists facing each other.

3 Bend your right arm close to your body.

4 Bend your left arm close to your body.

CHEST CROSSOVER

The Chest Crossover exercises the muscles of the upper back, arms, and chest.

This movement is the only one in which you move both arms away from each other and then back toward each other. You cross them at chest level.

ARM STATS

- Use the Chest Crossover with the Turn and the Alternating Wide-Step Tap Down.

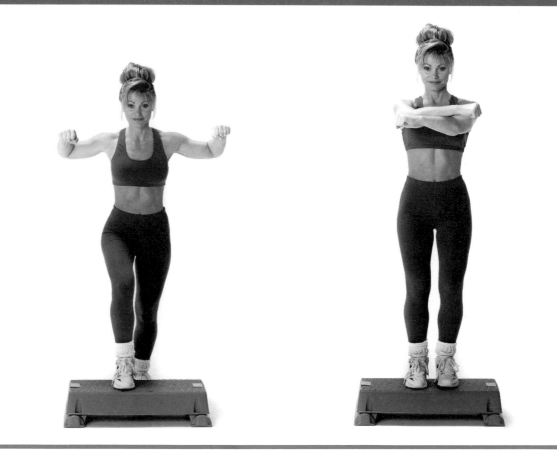

1 Start with your arms raised and bent at shoulder level, elbows out to the side, hands in a fist.

2 Keeping your elbows bent, move your arms toward each other at shoulder level and cross them.

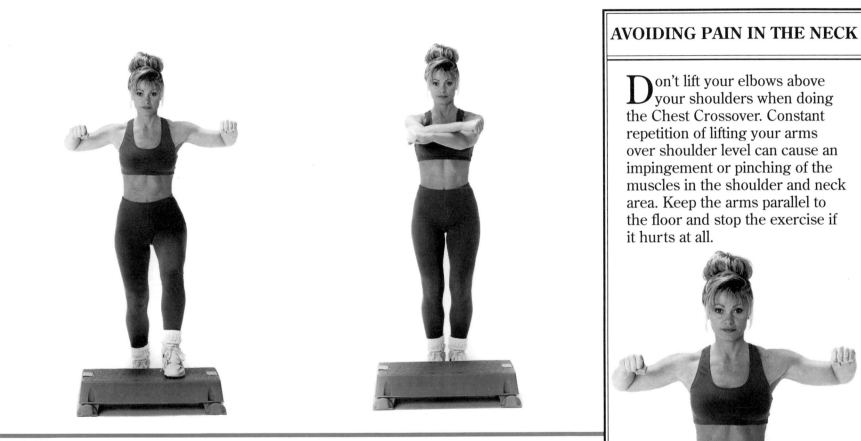

AVOIDING PAIN IN THE NECK

Don't lift your elbows above your shoulders when doing the Chest Crossover. Constant repetition of lifting your arms over shoulder level can cause an impingement or pinching of the muscles in the shoulder and neck area. Keep the arms parallel to the floor and stop the exercise if it hurts at all.

3 Keeping your bent arms parallel to the floor. Pull both arms open and back.

4 Pull your arms in and cross them at chest level.

*"Get to know your body—
use it or lose it."*

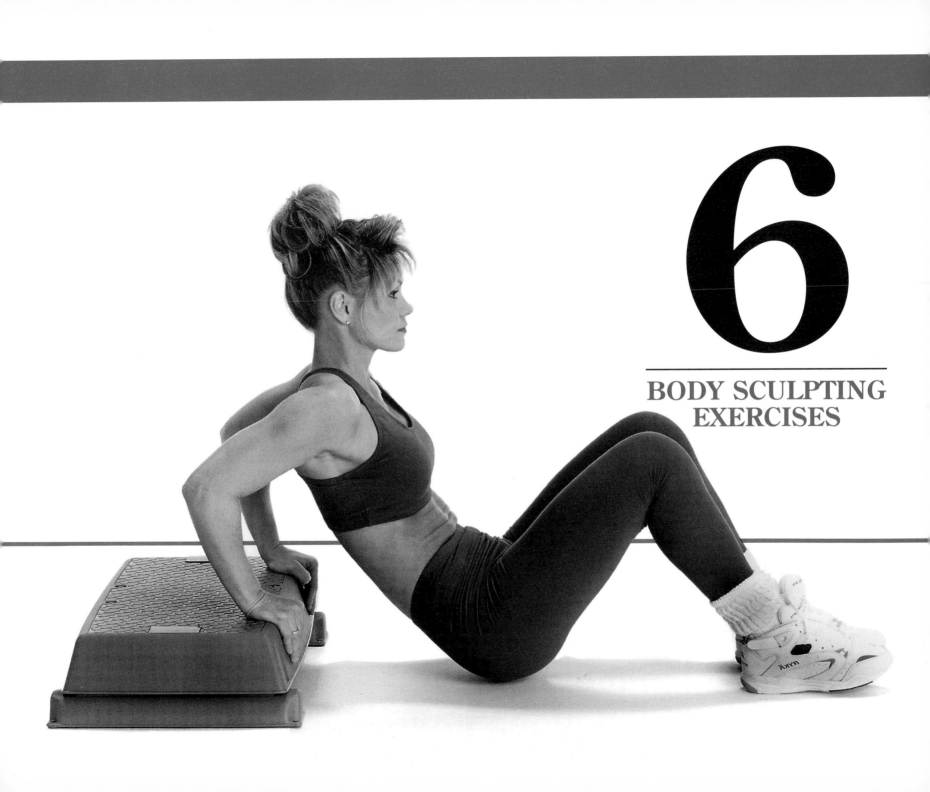

6

BODY SCULPTING EXERCISES

CHAPTER 6

BODY-SCULPTING EXERCISES

Body sculpting, or muscle conditioning, is one of the primary components of fitness. The American College of Sports Medicine recommends a muscle-conditioning workout twice a week. My program to increase muscle strength and endurance includes 8 to 12 repetitions of 8 to 10 exercises.

The body-sculpting exercises I've included in *Step Up Fitness* are designed to strengthen the muscles in both upper and lower body in order to increase lean muscle mass. Step Training automatically conditions the lower body, so to condition the upper body and assure a balanced workout, exercises that include the arms and torso must be added.

Using hand weights enhances the muscles and increases lean muscle mass.

Adding resistance increases the intensity of the muscle-conditioning exercises. My favorite resistance equipment is the rubber band. For more information on using the rubber band, read my *Original Rubber Band Workout* book.

The most commonly used type of resistance is hand weights. They're available in sporting goods and exercise equipment stores. I recommend that you begin with 1– to 3–pound weights. You can gradually increase the weights to 5 and 10 pounds as your muscle strength increases.

The Muscle Groups

The combination of a cardiovascular workout and body-sculpting exercises gives your whole body a balanced workout that benefits you inside as it makes your outside look great.

In body-sculpting, you use resistance in the form of the weights—the weight of your own body and in some cases hand weights. Resistance exercise is based on the principle of making your muscles work harder than they normally would.

Because they meet resistance, the muscles are strengthened as they expend more energy to achieve the goal.

Look at the picture on this page and locate the muscle groups. Each body-sculpting exercise strengthens specific muscle groups. Focus on these muscles as you perform the exercises.

Front of arm
(Biceps)

Upper back
(Rhomboids)

Shoulder
(Deltoid)

Back of arm
(Triceps)

Chest
(Pectoralis
major and
minor)

Stomach (Rectus
abdominus,
Obliquus
abdominus)

Hip flexor
(Iliopsoas)

Buttocks
(Gluteus
maximus and
minimus)

Front of thigh
(Quadriceps)

Back of thigh
(Hamstrings)

Outer thigh
(Gluteus
medius)

Inner thigh
(Adductors)

**Body sculpting is one of the
primary components of fitness.**

General Safety Reminders

- Do not lock your knees or bend them beyond a 90° angle.

- Do not hyperextend or arch the lower back.

- Contract the abdominal muscles to support the lower back.

- Keep proper body alignment at all times to avoid injuries.

- For floor exercises, place a mat or towel under your body for comfort.

- Above all, if you feel pain or discomfort, STOP the exercise.

Do NOT use weights if you have the following health conditions or problems:

- High blood pressure

- Pregnancy

- Arthritis or bursitis

- Heart disease

- Obesity

- Pain while exercising with weights

ALTERNATING LUNGE

This exercise conditions the muscles of your thighs and buttocks. By using the resistance of your own body weight, you lower and slowly push away from the platform.

Sculpting Stats

• Safety Tip: Don't bend your knees beyond a 90° angle.

• Repeat the exercise 10 times, alternating starting with your right and left legs.

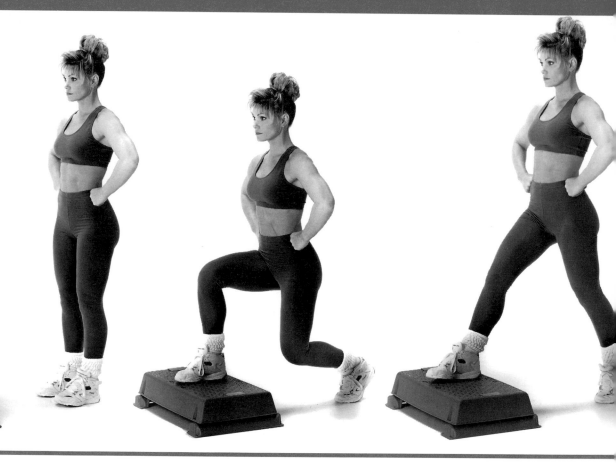

1 Stand about 3 feet away from the platform with your feet together, toes pointed straight ahead, hands in a fist and resting on your hips. Keep your pelvis tucked under, your spine straight, and your chin up.

2 Place one foot squarely on the platform and lunge forward. Never let your knee extend past your toes. Keep the back leg bent.

3 With your forward foot, slowly push yourself back off the platform and return your foot to the starting position. Repeat with the other leg.

PLIÉ

By placing one foot on the step and lifting your own body weight, you tone the adductor muscles in your inner thighs.

Sculpting Stats

• Safety Tip: Do not bend your knees beyond a 90° angle.

• Repeat the exercise 12 times with your right foot on the platform and 12 times with your left foot on the platform.

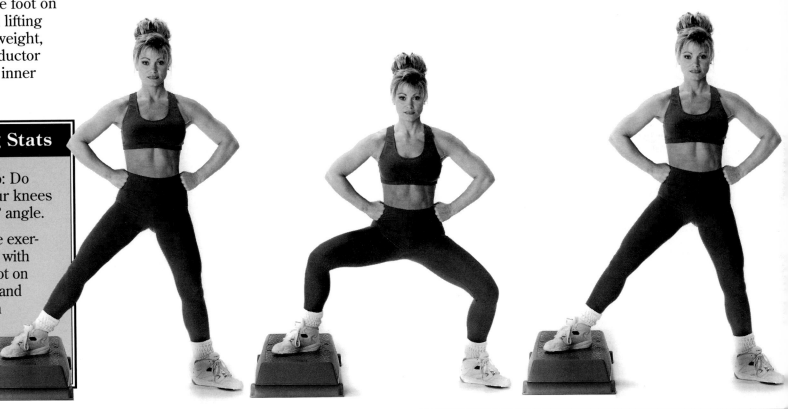

1 Stand about 3 feet away from the platform with the long edge to your right. Place your right foot on the center of the platform. Your left foot should remain on the floor on the right side of the platform. Hands are in a fist and rest on your hips.

2 Slowly bend both knees as you lower your body until your knees form 90° angles or less.

3 Slowly raise your body to a standing position.

SINGLE-LEG SQUAT

This exercise works the gluteus maximus and minimus muscles of your buttocks and upper thighs as you lower and lift your own body weight. Start with less depth to your bend and increase it as your muscles strengthen.

Sculpting Stats

- Safety Tips: Don't bend forward from the waist or bend the knee beyond a 90° angle.

- Repeat 8 times, then move to the other end of the platform and repeat 8 times with the other leg.

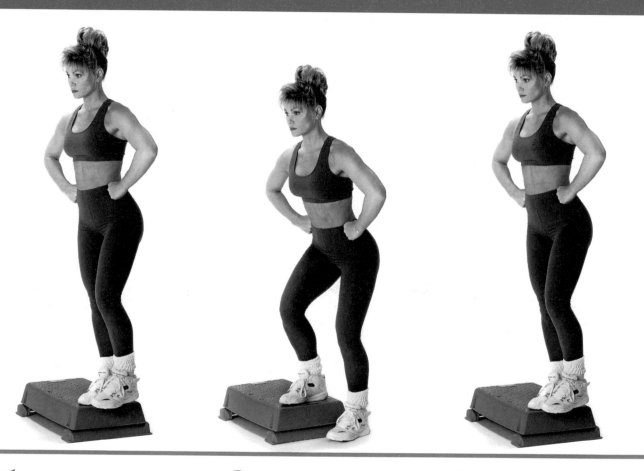

1 Stand with both feet together on one end of the platform. Hands are in a fist, resting on your hips.

2 Lift your outside foot and place it on the floor beside the short edge of the platform. Slowly lower your body, bending at the knees and hips but not at the waist. Don't bend your knees beyond a 90° angle.

3 Raise your body back to the standing position, bringing your outside foot up beside your supporting foot. Lift yourself by pressing through your heel.

OUTER LEG LIFT

In this exercise, you use your leg as a lever to work the gluteus medius muscle of the outer thigh. Start by raising your leg as high as you can, then increase the height as your strength improves.

Sculpting Stats

- Safety Tips: Keep your abdomen pulled in to support your lower back. Don't rotate your hips or knees.

- Repeat 8 times with each leg.

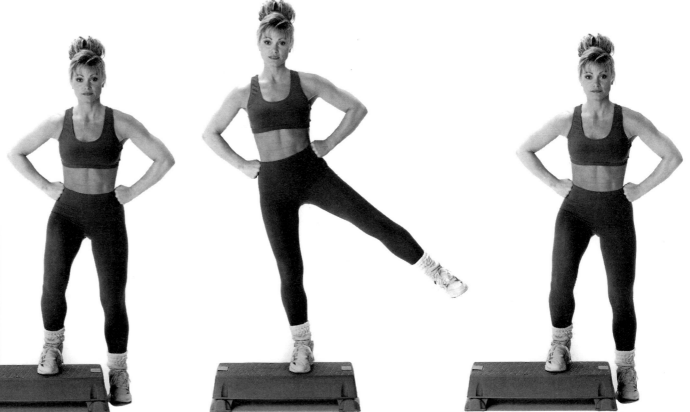

1 Stand with one foot on top of one end of the platform, the other on the floor beside the short edge of the platform. Hands are in a fist, resting on your hips.

2 Slowly lift the leg that is on the floor out to the side.

3 Slowly lower your leg to the starting position.

HAMSTRING HEEL PRESS

In this exercise, you work the quadriceps in the back of your thigh from a prone position. By pressing down on your heels and lifting your lower body from the platform, you strengthen and condition from the knee to the buttocks.

Sculpting Stats

- Safety Tip: Don't arch your back or lift it off the floor.
- Repeat 12 times.

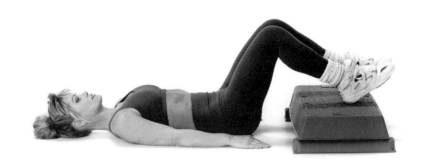

1 Lie on the floor with your back flat, both heels on the platform and both knees bent. Your arms should be straight down by your sides and your buttocks about a foot away from the platform.

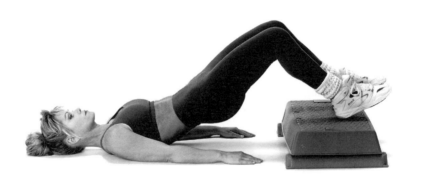

2 Keeping your knees bent and your upper back pressed against the floor, press your heels into the platform as you lift your buttocks slightly off the floor.

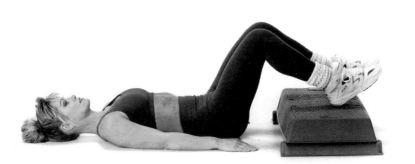

3 Slowly lower your buttocks to the floor.

PUSH-UP

The push-up is a great upper-body conditioner. Using the resistance of your own body weight, you work the muscles of the chest, shoulders, arms, and abdomen as you push up and lower your body.

Sculpting Stats

• Option: Support your lower torso with your legs extended as in a conventional pushup rather than on your knees.

• Repeat 10 times.

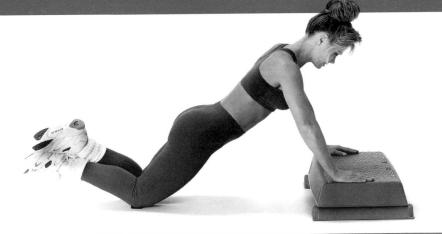

1 Beginning on your hands and knees with the long edge of the platform in front of you, place your hands on the platform about shoulder distance apart. Extend your arms so the line of your body makes a 45° angle with the floor. Your feet may come off the floor.

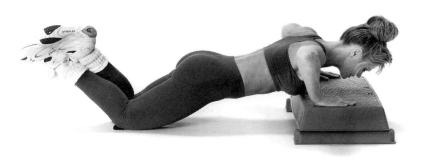

2 Slowly lower your upper body until your chest almost touches the platform. Keep a straight line of your body from your head to your knees.

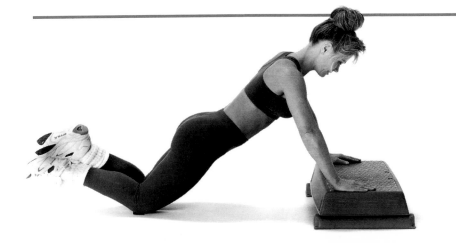

3 Slowly push yourself away from the platform with your arms, returning to the starting position.

TRICEPS PUSH-UP

This exercise works the much ignored muscle in the back of your arm—the sometimes sagging triceps. Using your body weight as resistance, with the platform behind you, lift and lower your body to strengthen and sculpt your triceps.

Sculpting Stats

- Safety Tips: Your elbows should not extend beyond a 90° angle. Don't lock your elbows as you lift your buttocks.

- Repeat 10 times.

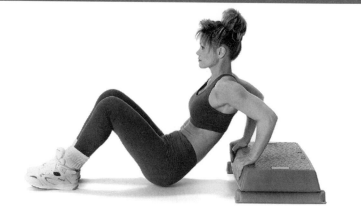

1 Sit on the floor facing away from the long edge of the platform. Keep your feet flat on the floor, and your knees bent at a 90° angle. Place both hands on the platform, palms facing down and your fingers wrapped gently around the front edge. Keep your back straight.

2 Lift your buttocks off the platform by pushing downward with your arms.

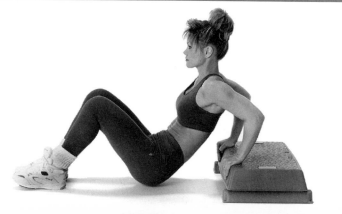

3 Slowly lower your buttocks to the floor.

REVERSE ARM LIFT

In this exercise, you lie on top of the platform and lift your arms to work the rhomboid and deltoid muscles in your upper back and shoulders.

1 Lie face down so that your body weight is completely supported by the platform. Extend your arms out to the side, bend your elbows to a 90° angle, and place your palms on the floor. Make sure your head is in line with your spine and that the platform is supporting your chest and abdomen.

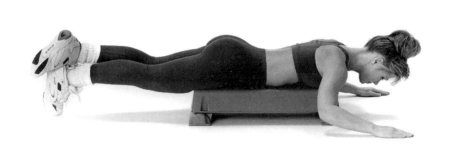

Sculpting Stats

- Safety Tips: Don't raise your head when you lift your arms. Don't arch your lower back.

- Repeat 12 times.

2 Lift your arms above your back, squeezing your shoulders together slightly.

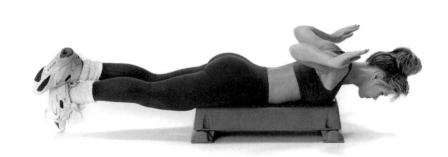

3 Lower your arms to the starting position.

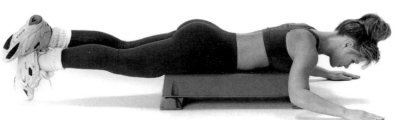

ABDOMINAL LIFT

From the prone position, feet on the platform, you lift your upper body to strengthen the rectus abdominus muscles of your abdomen.

Sculpting Stats

• Safety Tips: Inhale before you lift your shoulders, and exhale as you lift. Don't hold your breath. Don't arch your lower back. Hold your head in a neutral position by imagining a tennis ball held between your chin and chest.

• Repeat 12 times.

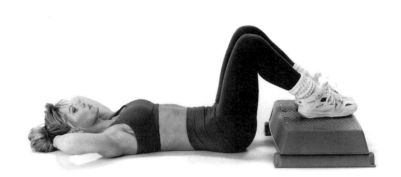

1 Lie flat on the floor, with your knees flexed and your feet on the platform. Put your hands behind your head with your elbows out to the sides.

2 Slowly lift your shoulders and arms off the floor.

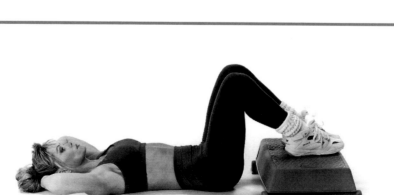

3 Lower your shoulders to their starting position on the floor.

ABDOMINAL CROSSOVER

Because one ankle is crossed over the knee of the opposite leg and you twist your body as you lift, this exercise works the obliquus abdominus muscles in your abdomen.

Sculpting Stats

- Safety Tips: Inhale before you raise your elbow and exhale as you lift. Keep your lower back on the floor and your head in a neutral position.

- Repeat 12 times on each side.

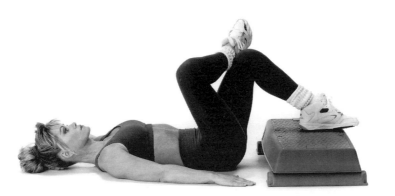

1 Lie on the floor with your back flat, left knee bent and your left foot on the platform. Rest your right ankle on your left knee. Place your left hand behind your head and extend your right arm next to your side.

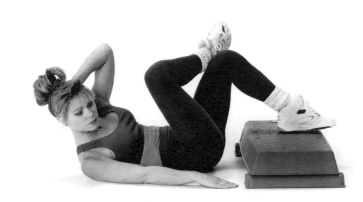

2 Lift your left elbow and bring it forward as if trying to touch your right knee.

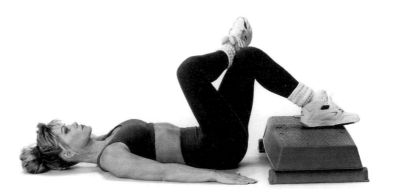

3 Return your left elbow to the starting position.

BICEPS CURL

This is the first exercise where you use hand weights for resistance. By lifting and lowering the weights, you work the biceps in the front of your arms.

Sculpting Stats

- Safety Tips: Keep your back straight and your head up.
- Repeat 12 times.

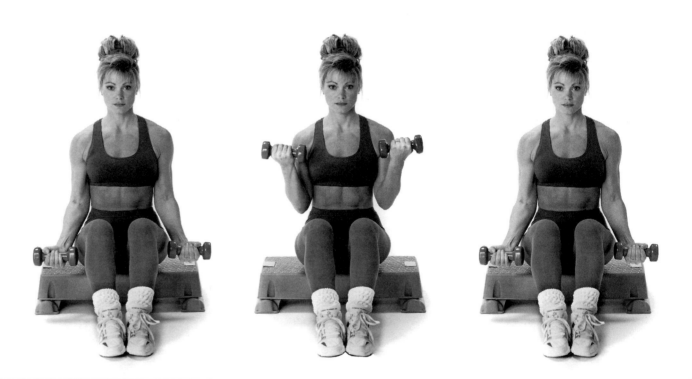

1 Sit on the center of the platform with your feet on the floor and your knees drawn up comfortably toward your chest. With your elbows at your sides, hold the weights gently with palms facing forward.

2 Slowly curl your forearms up toward your chest.

3 Slowly return your arms to the starting position.

OVERHEAD PRESS

In this exercise you lift hand weights overhead to work the deltoid muscles in your shoulders as well as the latissimus dorsi in your upper back.

Sculpting Stats

- Safety Tips: Pull in your abdomen as you lift your arms overhead. Don't arch your back.

- Repeat 12 times.

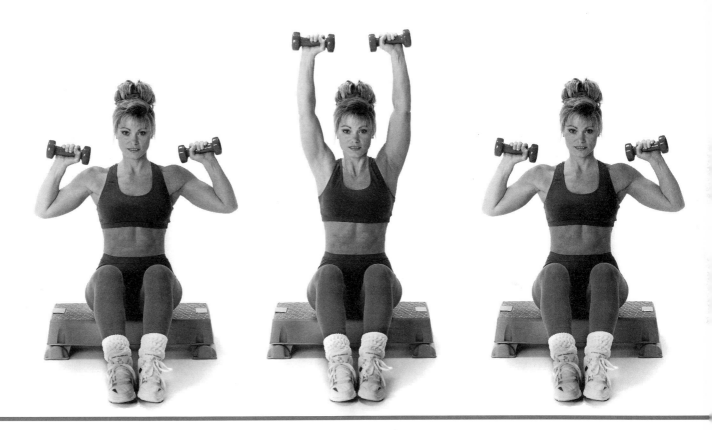

1 Sit on the center of the platform with your feet on the floor and your knees bent comfortably. Bend your arms so that your hands are next to your shoulders and your elbows are out to the side. Hold the weights gently, palms facing forward.

2 Raise both arms over your head, keeping the palms forward.

3 Slowly return both arms to the starting position.

"You have to make the decision to make fitness a part of your lifestyle."

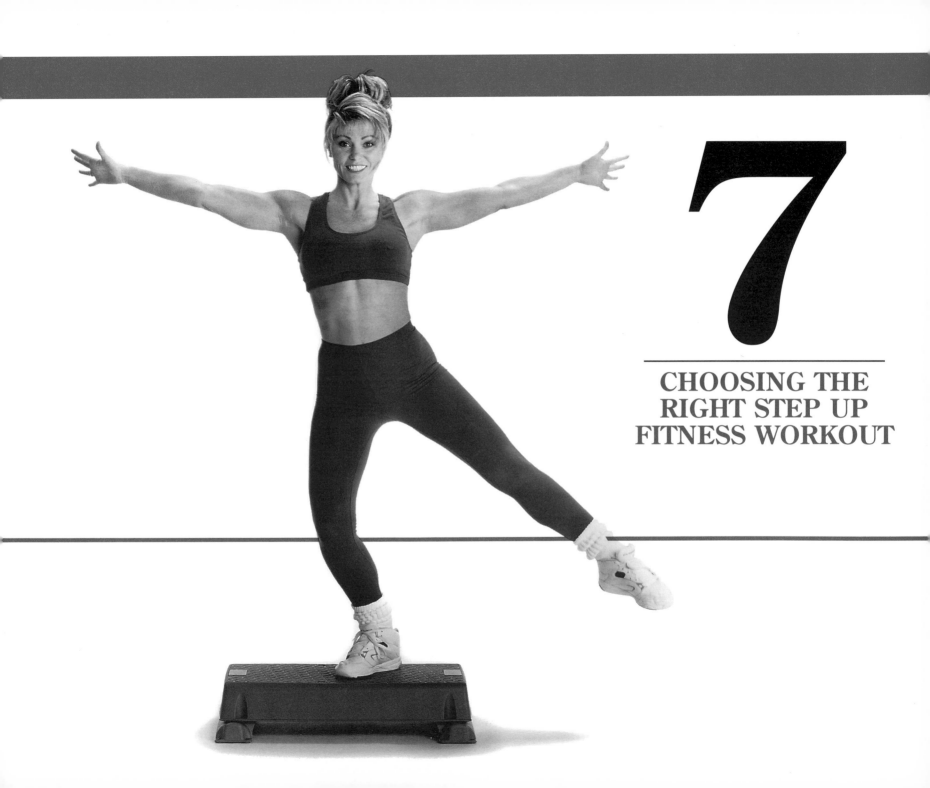

7

CHOOSING THE RIGHT STEP UP FITNESS WORKOUT

CHAPTER 7

CHOOSING THE RIGHT *STEP UP FITNESS* WORKOUT

Now that you've seen all the separate elements involved in *Step Up Fitness,* you can begin to see how all the parts add up to a well-rounded fitness workout.

Since each one of us is different, one workout can't possibly fit everyone. You don't have to look very far to realize that fitness levels are as different as the people who have them. Some of us are very fit, some are not so fit, and some of us aren't fit at all. We come in all different sizes, strengths, body types, and fitness levels. And because we differ, we all can't realistically participate in the same level of workout.

The solution is a good overall workout that can be adapted to match anyone's present ability yet permit them to move to a

Step Up Fitness lets you put together a fitness program that matches your fitness level.

The Right Height

Before doing the aerobic step test, estimate your present fitness level and set your platform height as described.

- FAIR: Raise the platform 6 inches from the floor.

- GOOD: Raise the platform 8 inches.

- EXCELLENT: Raise the platform 12 inches.

Note: If you are short, even if you are in excellent shape, never raise the platform so high that your knee bends more than 90 degrees.

higher level as they improve. And that's just what my Step Training workouts do. They provide for different fitness levels, so you can begin to work out at once, regardless of the condition you're in. *Step Up Fitness* lets you put together a fitness workout that matches your fitness level. And regardless of the condition you're in now, the whole idea behind Step Training is to improve. Whatever level you're at now, you won't be there long.

I've designed workouts for three different fitness levels: one for beginners, one for intermediates, and one for those who are advanced. To select the workout that suits you best right now, all you have to do is to evaluate your present physical condition.

When you evaluate your fitness level, underestimate rather than overestimate. It's a lot easier to work up to higher levels than it is to struggle with a workout that's unnecessarily strenuous. Start where you're comfortable. And, of course, if you have any questions regarding your ability to participate in an active conditioning workout, consult your physician first.

Aerobic Step Test

To determine your current fitness level, you can give yourself a simple test. What it does is to raise your heart rate and breathing rate so that you can estimate your overall cardiopulmonary condition. This is not a controlled stress test, but it will give you an approximation of your present condition.

Again, a lower guess is better than over-estimating your condition if you're not sure.

Stand in the front starting position. Begin with your right foot and repeat the Basic Right pattern for 1½ minutes. Then repeat the Basic Left pattern for 1½ minutes.

Stop after you've completed the 3-minute sequence and immediately note your breathing rate.

As a rule of thumb, if you can carry on a normal conversation without puffing or gasping for air, you're in pretty good shape and should be able to comfortably complete any of the three *Step Up Fitness* workouts. If your breathing is labored, begin with Workout One or Two. If you puff or gasp for air, start with Workout One.

I recommend that anyone who is new to Step Training, regardless of physical condition, begin with Workout One to become thoroughly familiar with the step patterns, the rhythm, and the upper body moves. Once they are second nature, you can move on to the intensity level suited to your condition.

"Step Up Fitness *lets you put together a fitness workout that matches your fitness level.* **"**

Ready, Set, Go!

If you have worked carefully through all the Step Patterns, Arm Movements and Body-Sculpting Exercises, you should have a good understanding of how to follow the workouts in this section. Each of the three workouts has one box that tells you the schedule and routine and another that tells you what to do on each exercise day.

After you have chosen the workout for your fitness level, let the photographs guide you through the step pattern and body-sculpting sequences. If you get confused about any of the patterns or exercises, refer to the page number given for complete instructions.

Whenever you feel you need a break in the intensity of the workout or need to regain orientation, continue your workout on the floor instead of on the platform, or, if you are performing Arm Movements, relax your arms and put your hands on your hips until you recover.

WORKOUT ONE: BEGINNER

In the *Step Up Fitness* Beginner Workout, you exercise from 30 to 35 minutes a day, three days a week. The workout begins with warm-up and stretching and ends with cool-down and stretching. Warm-up and cool-down take 10 to 15 minutes, Step Training occupies 10 minutes, and 10 minutes are devoted to body sculpting.

Schedule & Routine

Days of the week	3
Warm up/Stretch	5–8 minutes
Step	10 minutes
Sculpt	10 minutes
Cool down/Stretch	5–8 minutes
Total time	30–35 minutes

Days 1, 3, 5: Exercise
Days 2, 4: Rest

STEP PATTERN SEQUENCE

BASIC RIGHT
(p. 44)

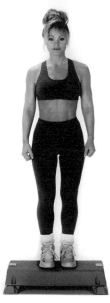

BASIC LEFT *(p. 46)*

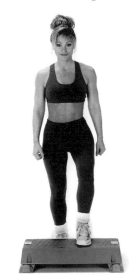
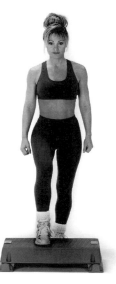

STEP PATTERNS

Each Day

On each exercise day:

1. Warm up and stretch (Chapter 3).

2. Perform each step pattern 8 times.

3. Perform the entire sequence of step patterns once.

4. Do each body-sculpting exercise the number of times indicated.

5. Cool down and stretch (Chapter 3).

WIDE STEP *(p. 48)*

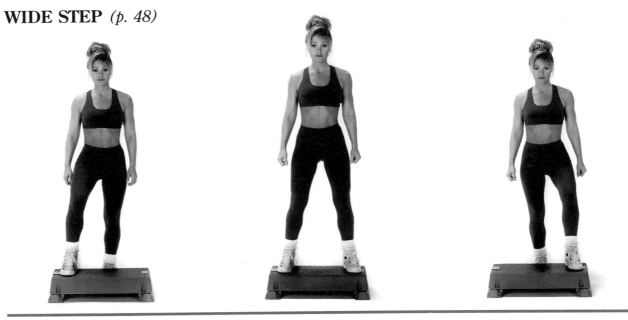

ALTERNATING TAP DOWN *(p. 50)*

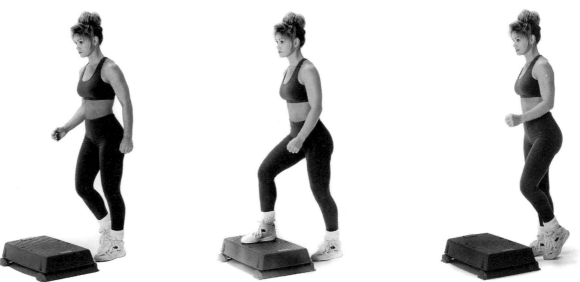

WORKOUT ONE: BEGINNER

TURN *(p. 62)*

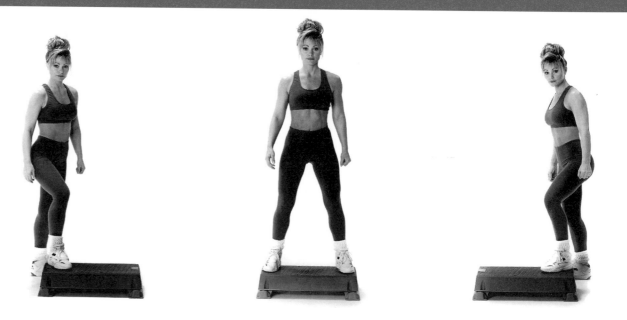

TAP UP/TAP DOWN *(p. 66)*

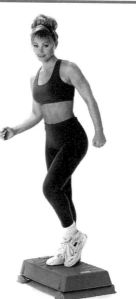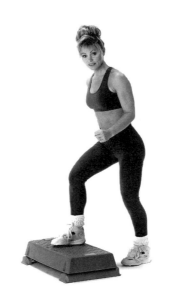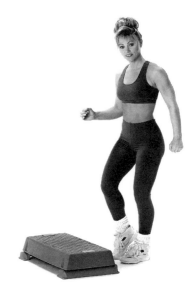

STEP PATTERNS

REPEATER KNEE
LIFT *(p. 68)*

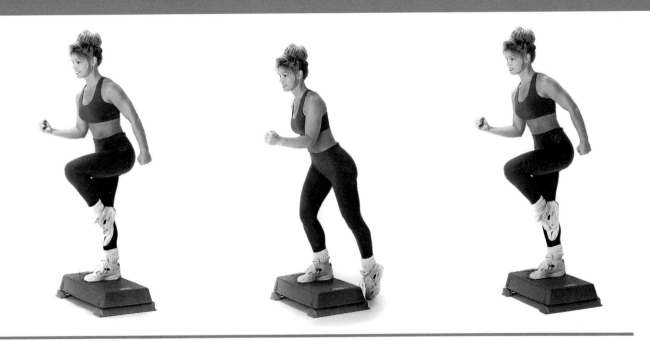

REPEATER HEEL
LIFT *(p. 68)*

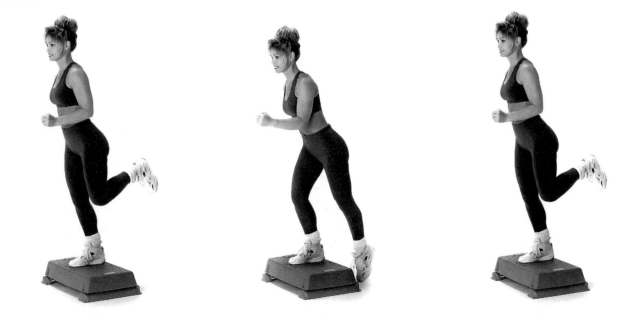

WORKOUT ONE: BEGINNER

REPEATER LEG LIFT
(p. 68)

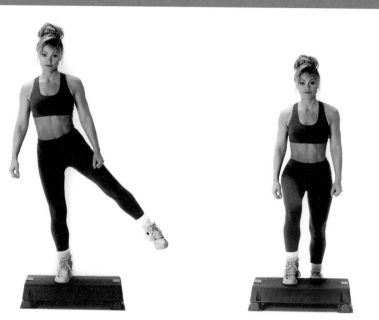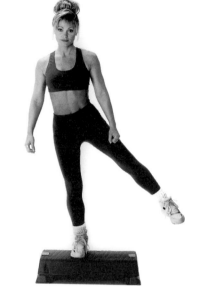

**ALTERNATING TAP
UP** *(p. 52)*

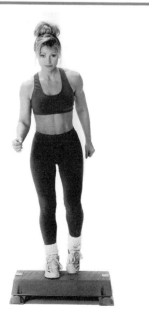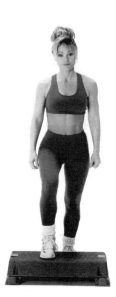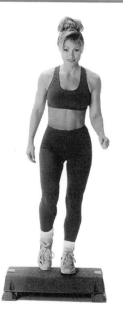

STEP PATTERNS

**ALTERNATING KNEE
LIFT** *(p. 56)*

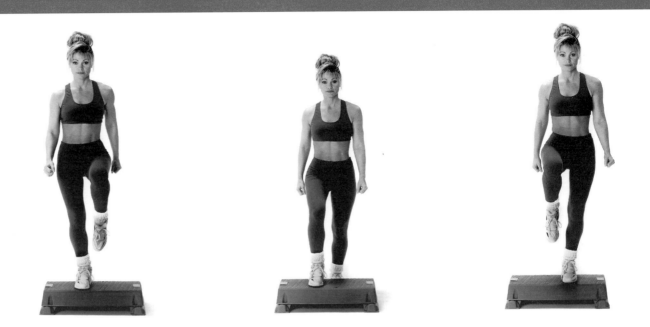

**ALTERNATING LEG
LIFT** *(p. 58)*

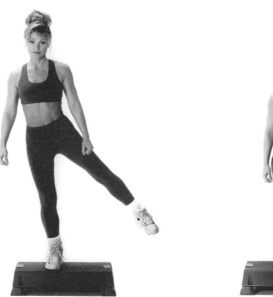
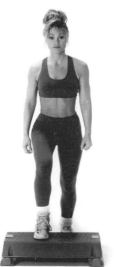
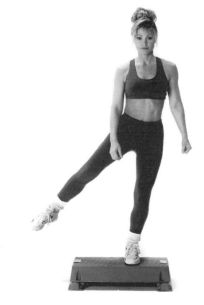

WORKOUT ONE: BEGINNER

ALTERNATING HEEL LIFT *(p. 60)*

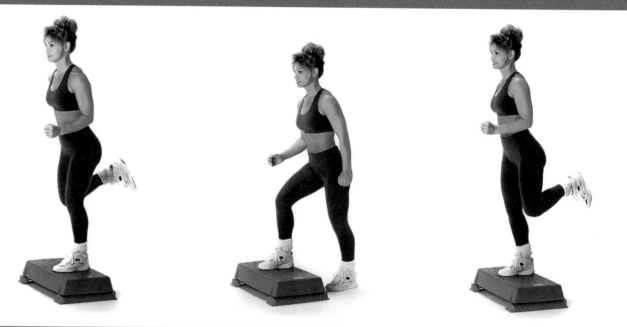

ALTERNATING WIDE-STEP TAP DOWN *(p. 54)*

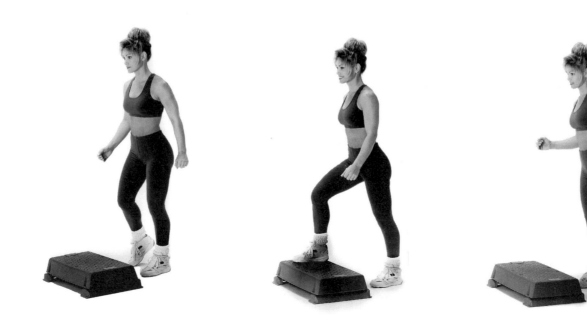

STEP PATTERNS

OVER THE TOP
(p. 64)

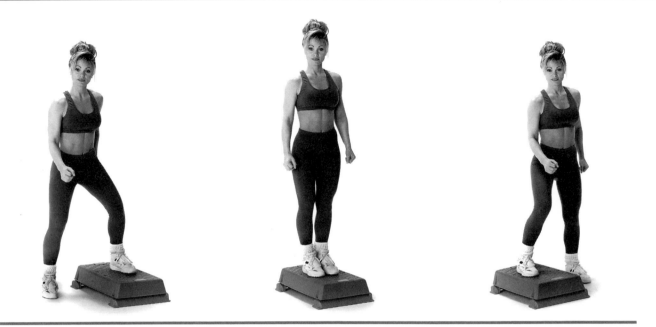

STRADDLE DOWN
(p. 72)

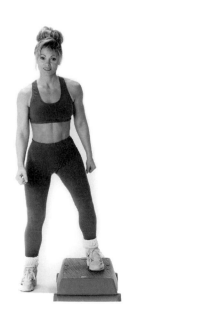
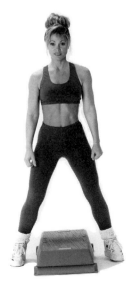
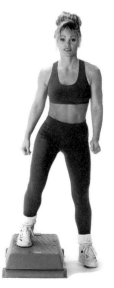

WORKOUT ONE: BEGINNER

**ALTERNATING TAP
UP/STRADDLE DOWN**
(p. 74)

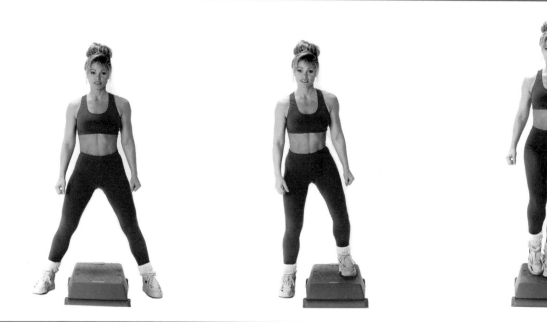

ACROSS THE TOP
(p. 76)

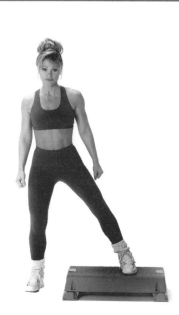
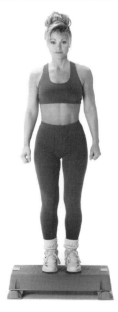
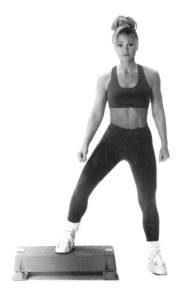

BODY-SCULPTING EXERCISES

**ALTERNATING
LUNGE** *(p. 70)*

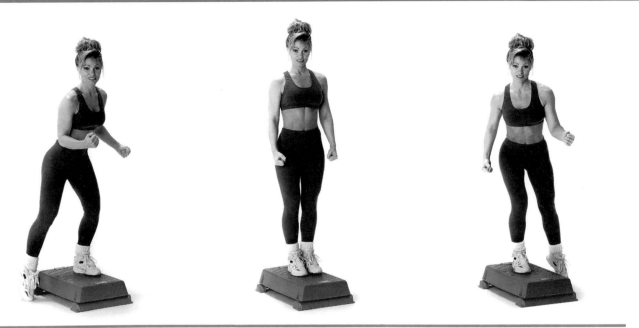

BODY-SCULPTING SEQUENCE

**HAMSTRING HEEL
PRESS** *(p. 102)*
12 repetitions

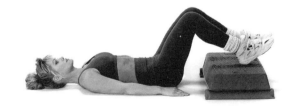 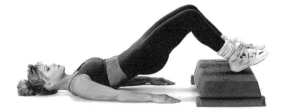

WORKOUT ONE: BEGINNER

**ALTERNATING
LUNGE** *(P. 98)*

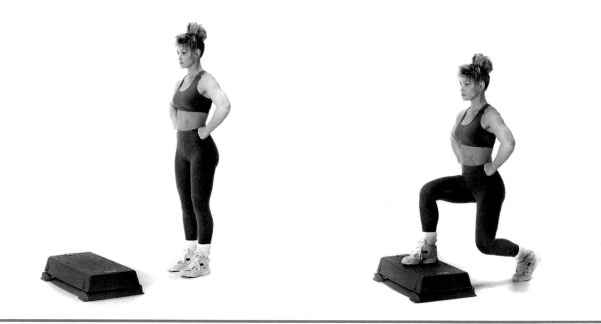

PLIÉ *(p. 99)*
12 repetitions

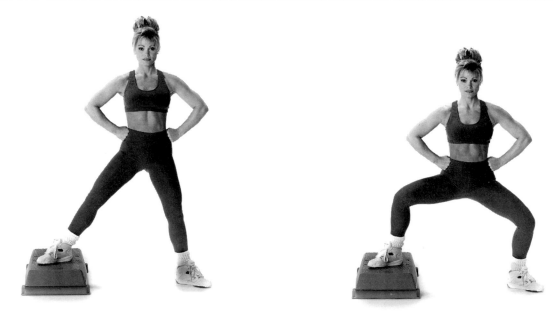

BODY-SCULPTING EXERCISES

OUTER LEG LIFT

(p. 101) 8 repetitions

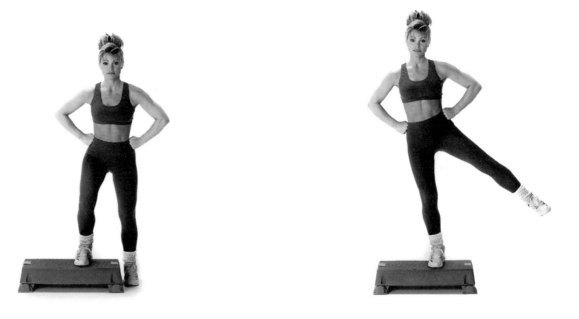

TRICEPS PUSH-UP

(p. 104) 10 repetitions

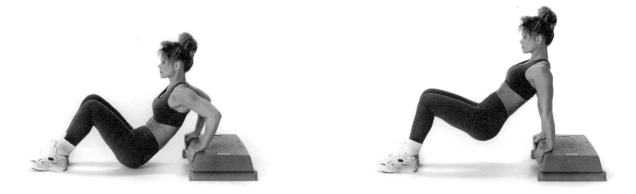

WORKOUT ONE: BEGINNER

OVERHEAD PRESS
(p. 109) 10 repetitions

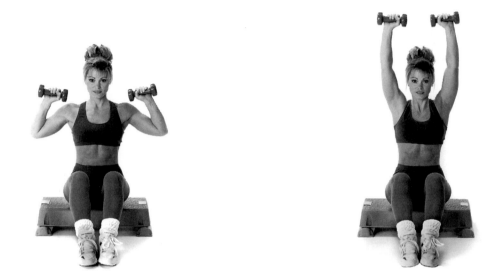

BICEPS CURL
(p. 108) 12 repetitions

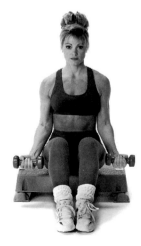
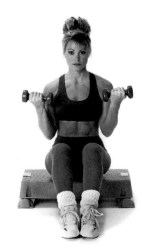

BODY-SCULPTING EXERCISES

REVERSE ARM LIFT
(p. 105) 12 repititions

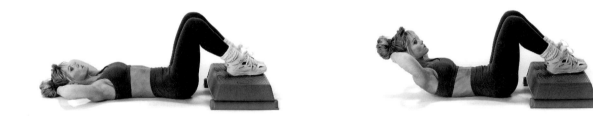

ABDOMINAL LIFT
(p. 106) 12 repetitions

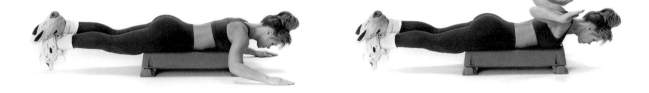

ABDOMINAL CROSSOVER *(p. 107)*
12 repetitions

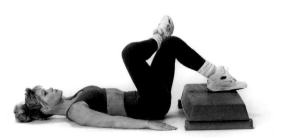
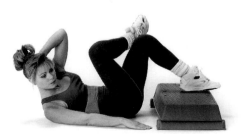

WORKOUT TWO: INTERMEDIATE

In the *Step Up Fitness* Intermediate Workout, you exercise from 40 to 45 minutes a day, three days a week. The workout begins with warm-up and stretching and ends with cool-down and stretching for 10 to 15 minutes. Step Training occupies 20 minutes, and 10 minutes of the workout are for body sculpting.

Schedule & Routine
Days of the week 3
Warm up/Stretch 5–8 minutes
Step 20 minutes
Sculpt 10 minutes
Cool down/Stretch 5–8 minutes
Total time 40–45 minutes
Days 1, 3, 5: Exercise Days 2, 4: Rest

STEP PATTERN SEQUENCE

BASIC RIGHT *(p. 44)* **WITH BICEPS CURL** *(p. 82)*

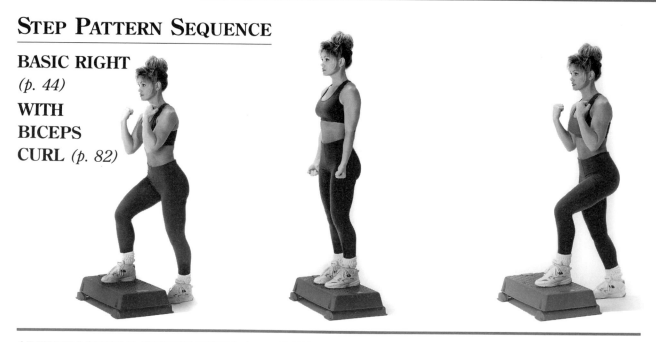

ALTERNATING KNEE LIFT *(p. 56)* **WITH OVERHEAD PRESS** *(p. 86)*

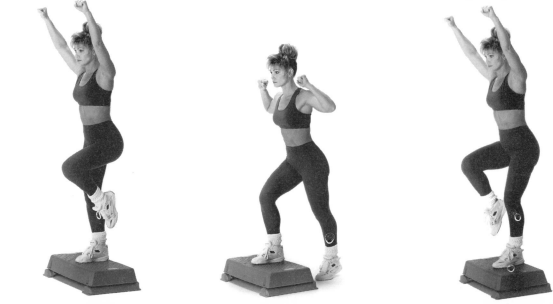

STEP PATTERNS

Each Day

On each exercise day:

1. Warm up and stretch (Chapter 3).

2. Perform each step pattern with arm movements 8 times.

3. Repeat the entire step pattern sequence 4 times.

4. Do each body-sculpting exercise the number of times indicated.

5. Cool down and stretch (Chapter 3).

BASIC LEFT *(p. 46)* WITH SHOULDER PUNCH *(p. 84)*

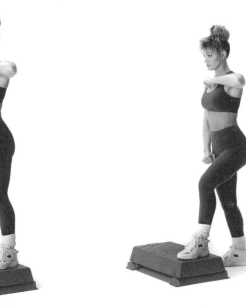

WIDE STEP *(p. 48)* WITH ALTERNATING UPRIGHT ROW *(p. 89)*

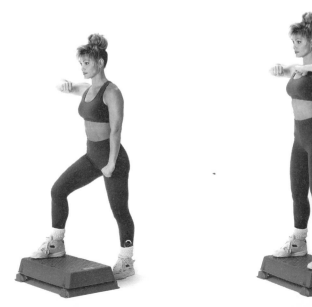

WORKOUT TWO: INTERMEDIATE

**ALTERNATING
WIDE-STEP TAP
DOWN** *(p. 54)*
**WITH ALTERNATING
UPRIGHT ROW**
(p. 89)

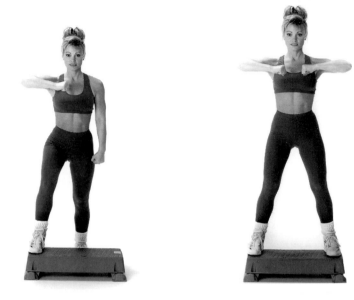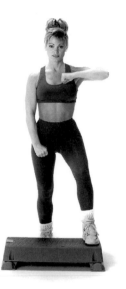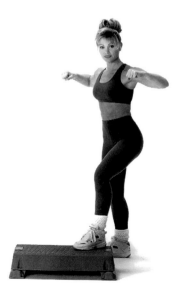

TURN *(p. 62)*
**WITH CHEST
CROSSOVER** *(p. 92)*

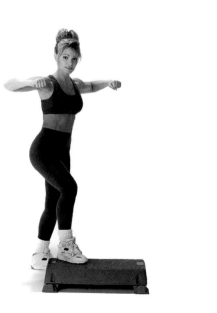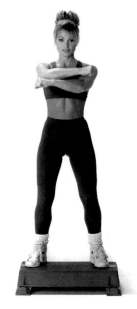

STEP PATTERNS

**ALTERNATING TAP
DOWN** *(p. 50)*
WITH BICEPS CURL
(p. 82)

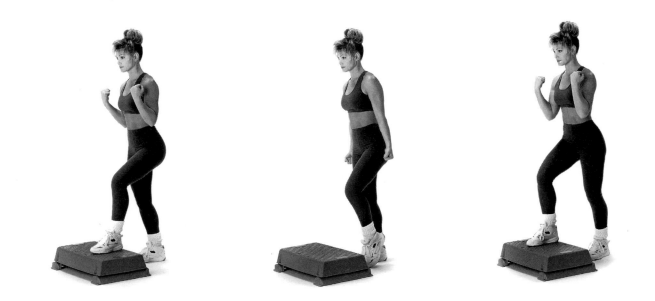

OVER THE TOP
(p. 64) **WITH OVER-
HEAD PRESS** *(p. 86)*

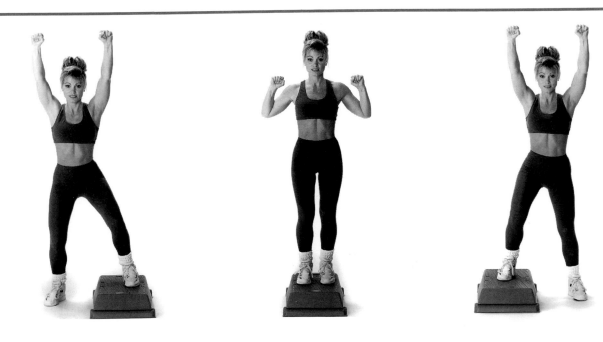

WORKOUT TWO: INTERMEDIATE

REPEATER KNEE LIFT *(p. 68)* **OVER THE TOP** *(p. 64)* **WITH SHOULDER PUNCH** *(p. 84)*

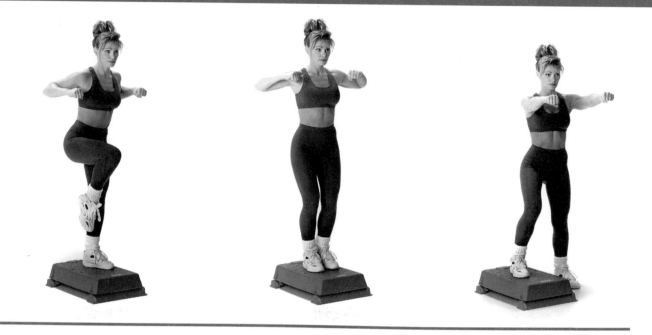

STRADDLE DOWN *(p. 72)* **ALTERNATING KNEE LIFT** *(p. 56)* **WITH OVERHEAD PRESS** *(p. 86)*

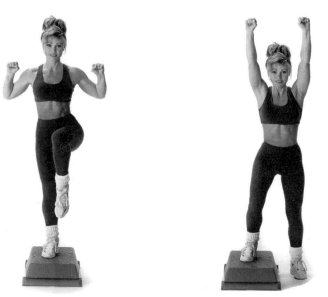
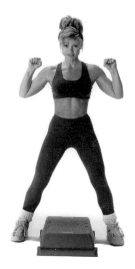

STEP PATTERNS

ALTERNATING LUNGE *(p. 70)* **WITH ALTERNATING SHOULDER PUNCH** *(p. 85)*

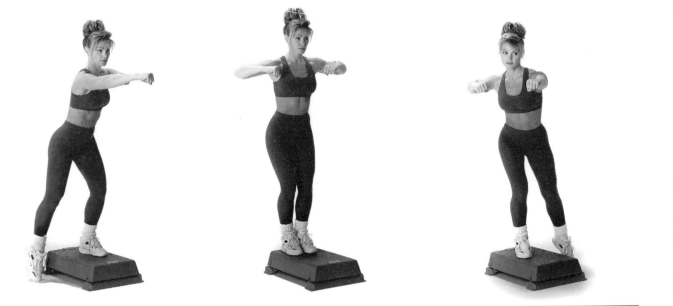

STRADDLE DOWN *(p. 72)* **WITH ALTERNATING BICEPS CURL** *(p. 83)*

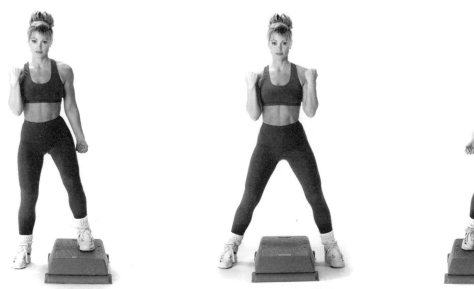
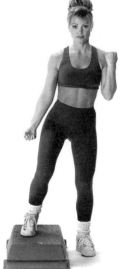

WORKOUT TWO: INTERMEDIATE

**ALTERNATING
KNEE LIFT** *(p. 56)*
STRADDLE DOWN
(p. 72) **WITH
TRICEPS KICK BACK**
(p. 90)

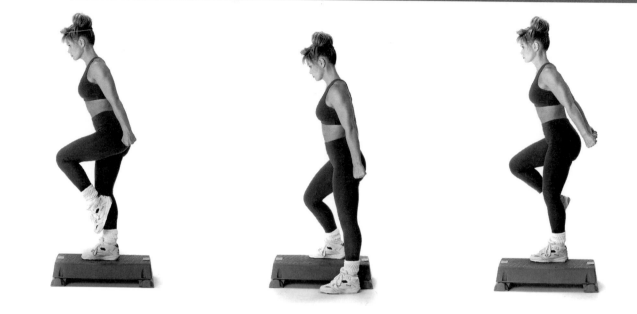

**ALTERNATING
LUNGE** *(p. 70)*
**WITH ALTERNATING
SHOULDER PUNCH**
(p. 85)

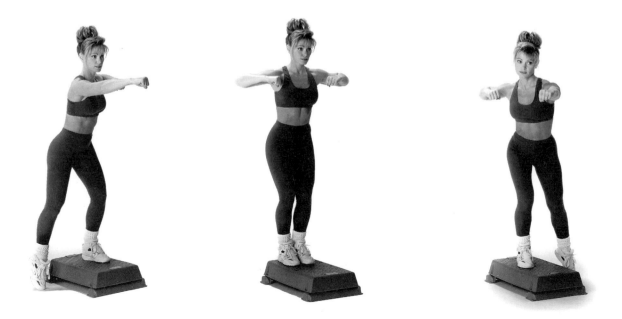

STEP PATTERNS

STRADDLE DOWN
(p. 72) **WITH**
ALTERNATING
BICEPS CURL *(p. 83)*

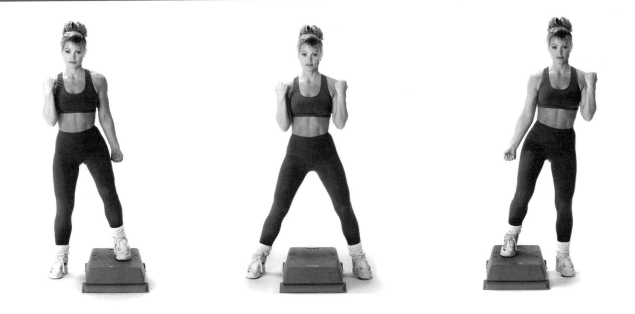

REPEATER LEG LIFT
(p. 68) **WITH BICEPS**
CURL *(p. 82)*

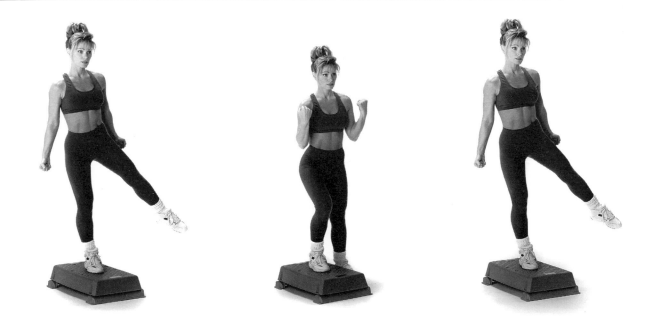

WORKOUT TWO: INTERMEDIATE

**ALTERNATING TAP
DOWN** *(p. 50)* **WITH
BICEPS CURL** *(p. 82)*

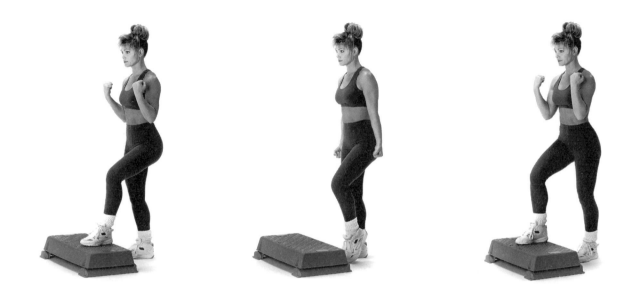

WIDE STEP *(p. 48)*
**WITH ALTERNATING
UPRIGHT ROW**
(p. 89)

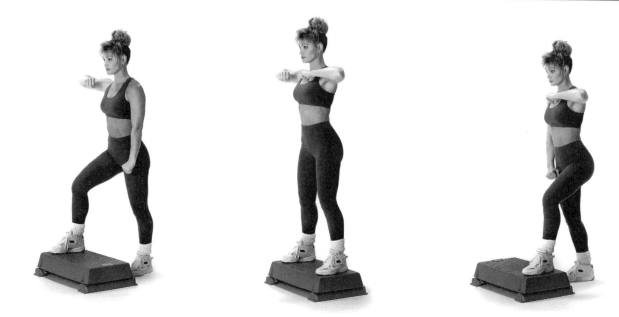

STEP PATTERNS

BASIC LEFT *(p. 46)*
WITH ALTERNATING
BICEPS CURL *(p. 83)*

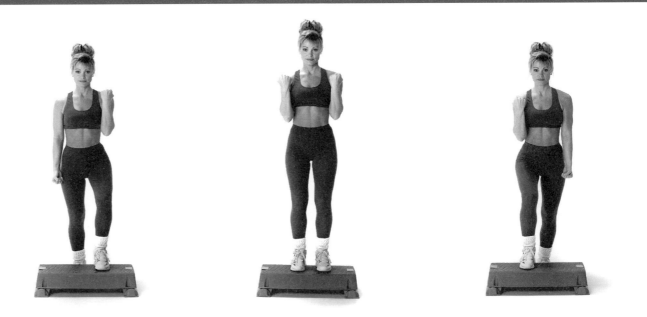

REPEATER HEEL
LIFT *(p. 68)* **WITH**
TRICEPS KICK BACK
(p. 90)

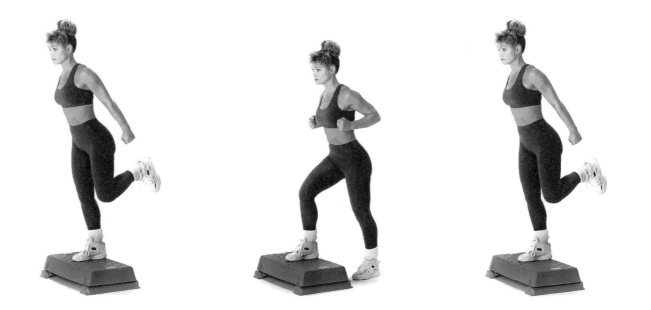

WORKOUT TWO: INTERMEDIATE

BASIC RIGHT *(p. 44)*
WITH UPRIGHT ROW
(p. 88)

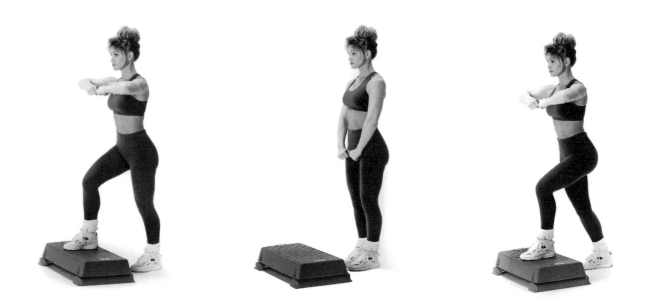

**REPEATER KNEE
LIFT** *(p. 68)* **WITH
OVERHEAD PRESS**
(p. 86)

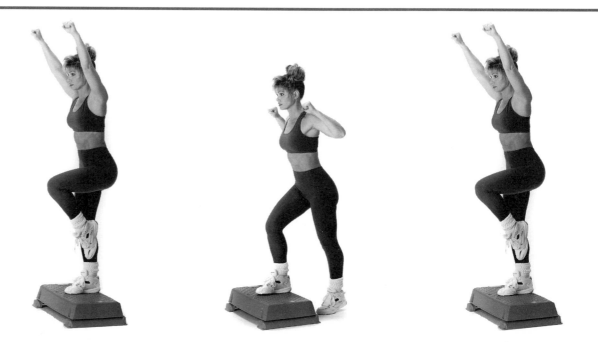

STEP PATTERNS

ACROSS THE TOP *(p. 76)* **WITH OVERHEAD PRESS** *(p. 86)*

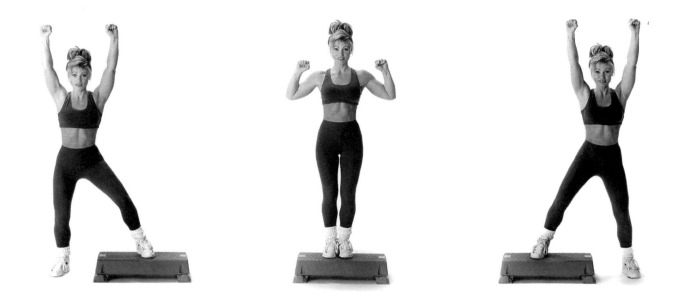

TAP UP/TAP DOWN *(p. 66)* **WITH ALTERNATING BICEPS CURL** *(p. 83)*

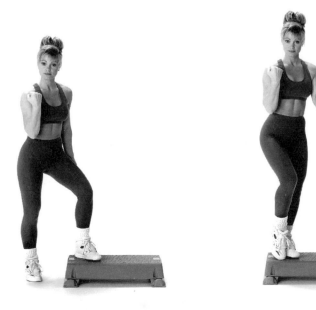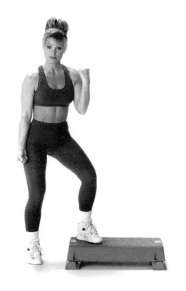

WORKOUT TWO: INTERMEDIATE

ACROSS THE TOP
(p. 76) **TAP UP/TAP DOWN** *(p. 66)* **WITH OVERHEAD PRESS**
(p. 86)

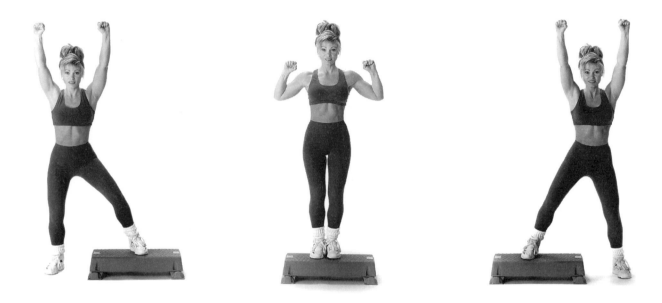

BODY-SCULPTING SEQUENCE

ALTERNATING LUNGE *(p. 98)*
16 repetitions

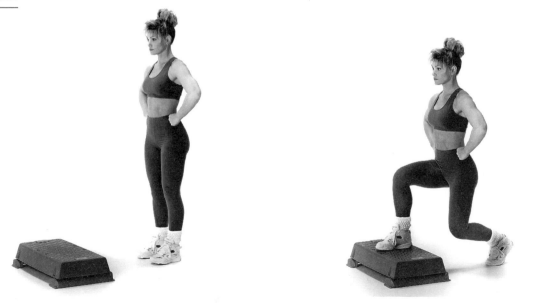

BODY-SCULPTING EXERCISES

PLIÉ *(p. 99)*
16 repetitions

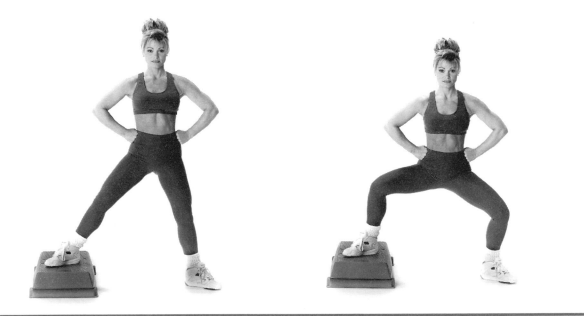

TRICEPS PUSH-UP
(p. 104) 16 repetitions

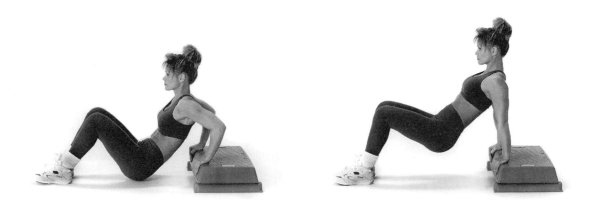

WORKOUT TWO: INTERMEDIATE

PUSH-UP *(p. 103)*
10 repetitions

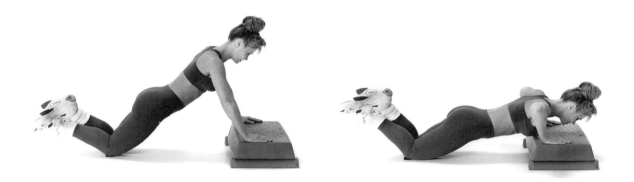

REVERSE ARM LIFT
(p. 105) 16 repetitions

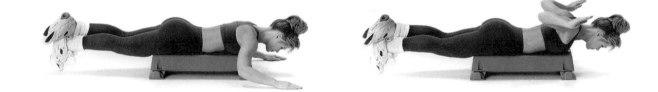

BICEPS CURL
(p. 108) 10 repetitions

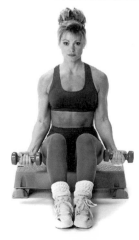
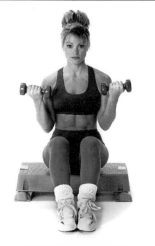

BODY-SCULPTING EXERCISES

OVERHEAD PRESS
(p. 109) 10 repetitions

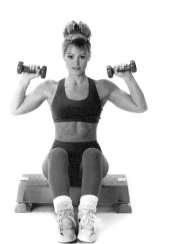
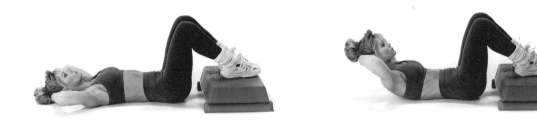

ABDOMINAL LIFT
(p. 106) 25 repetitions

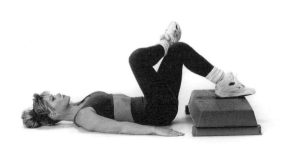

ABDOMINAL CROSSOVER *(p. 107)*
10 repetitions

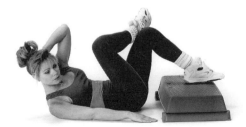

WORKOUT THREE: ADVANCED DAYS 1, 3 & 5

In the *Step Up Fitness* Advanced Workout, you exercise from 40 to 45 minutes a day, five days a week. Three of the five days are devoted to Step Training, with warm-up and stretch and cool-down and stretch periods. On the alternating two days, body sculpting occupies 30 minutes, again with warm-up and stretch and cool-down and stretch.

Schedule & Routine

Days of the week
5
Warm up/Stretch 5–8 minutes
Step or Sculpt 30 minutes
Cool down/Stretch 5–8 minutes
Total time 40–45 minutes

Days 1, 3, 5: Step Training
Days 2, 4: Body Sculpting

DAYS 1, 3, 5 STEP PATTERN SEQUENCE

1. BASIC RIGHT *(p. 44)* WITH UPRIGHT ROW *(p. 88)*
8 repetitions

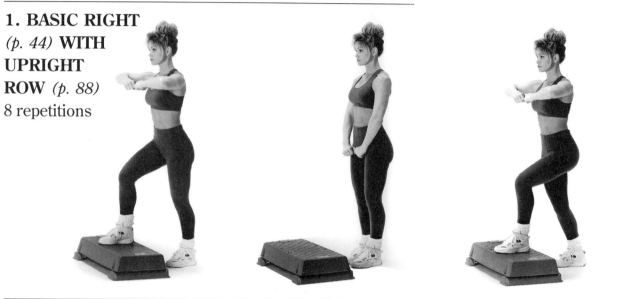

2. ALTERNATING REPEATER KNEE LIFT *(p. 68)* WITH OVERHEAD PRESS *(p. 86)* 1 repetition

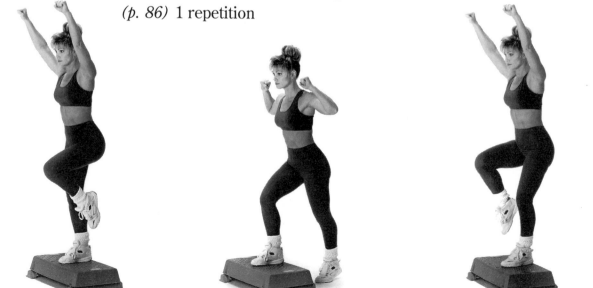

STEP PATTERNS

3. BASIC LEFT *(p. 46)* WITH ALTERNATING BICEPS CURL *(p. 83)*

8 repetitions   Repeat Exercises 1–3 in sequence 4 times.

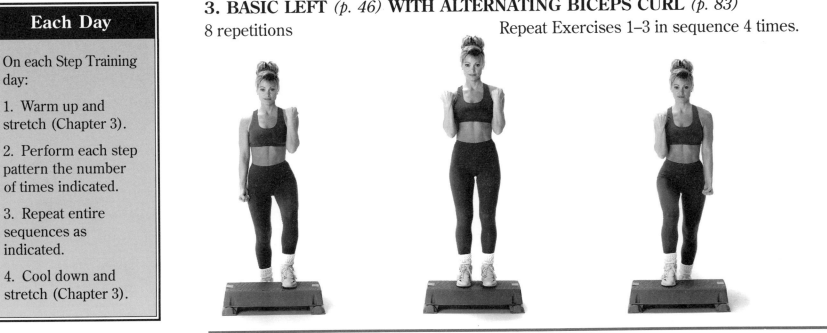

4. ALTERNATING LEG LIFT *(p. 58)* WITH TRICEPS KICK BACK *(p. 90)*

4 repetitions

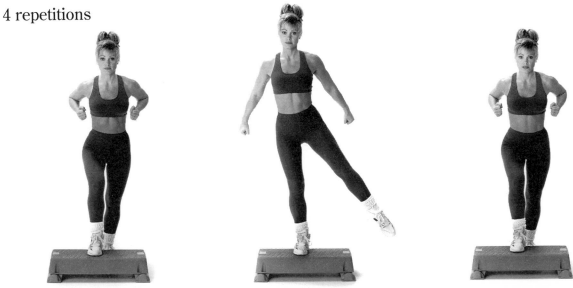

WORKOUT THREE: ADVANCED DAYS 1, 3 & 5

5. OVER THE TOP
(p. 64) **WITH**
OVERHEAD PRESS
(p. 86) 7 repetitions

Repeat Exercises 4–5 in
sequence 4 times.

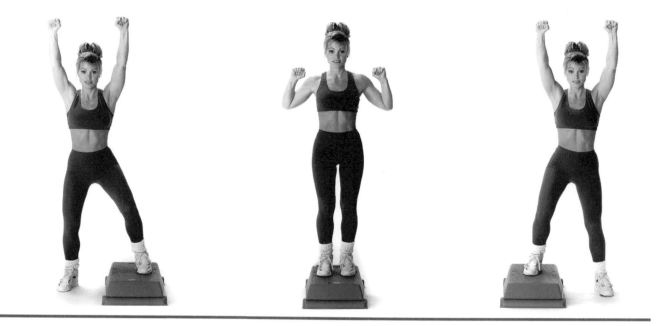

6. TURN *(p. 62)* **WITH**
CHEST CROSSOVER
(p. 92) 8 repetitions

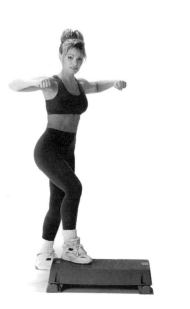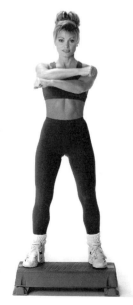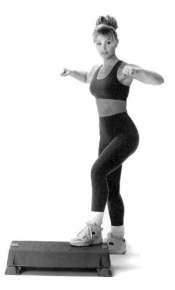

STEP PATTERNS

7. ALTERNATING HEEL LIFT *(p. 60)* WITH TRICEPS KICK BACK *(p. 90)*

4 repetitions

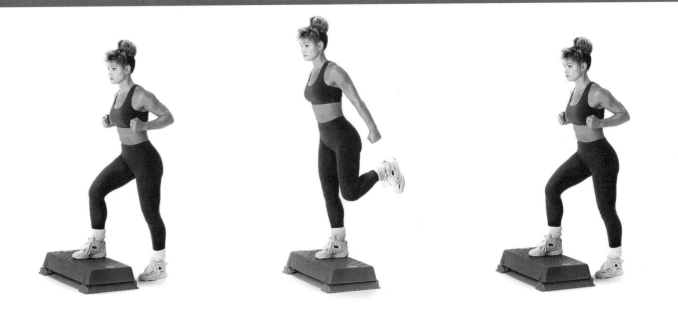

8. TURN *(p. 62)* WITH CHEST CROSSOVER

(p. 92) 7 repetitions

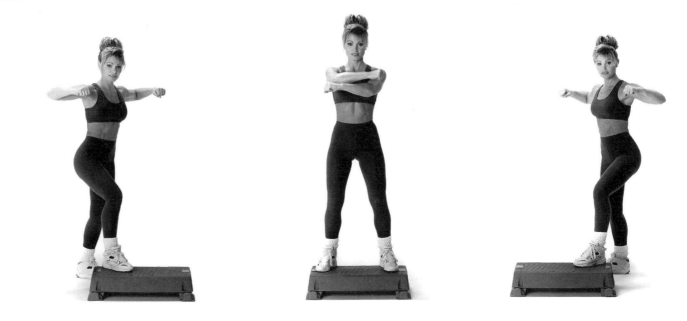

WORKOUT THREE: ADVANCED DAYS 1, 3 & 5

9. WIDE STEP *(p. 48)*
WITH ALTERNATING
UPRIGHT ROW
(p. 89) 8 repetitions

Repeat exercises 6–8 in
sequence 4 times.

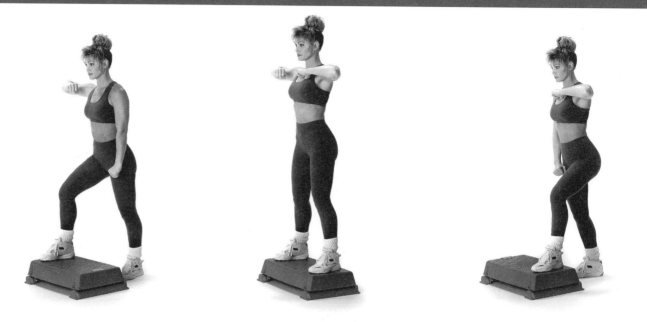

10. ALTERNATING
KNEE LIFT *(p. 56)*
WITH OVERHEAD
PRESS *(p. 86)*
8 repetitions

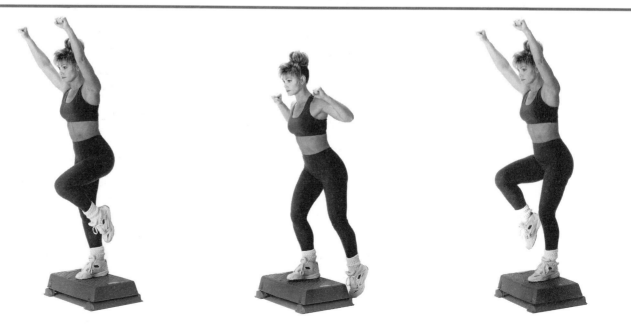

STEP PATTERNS

11. ALTERNATING REPEATER KNEE LIFT *(p. 56)* WITH SHOULDER PUNCH
(p. 84) 1 repetition

Repeat exercises 9–11 in sequence 4 times.

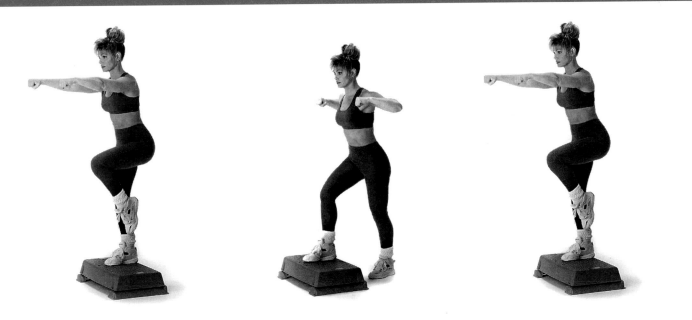

12. BASIC RIGHT *(p. 44)* WITH BICEPS CURL *(p. 82)*
3 repetitions

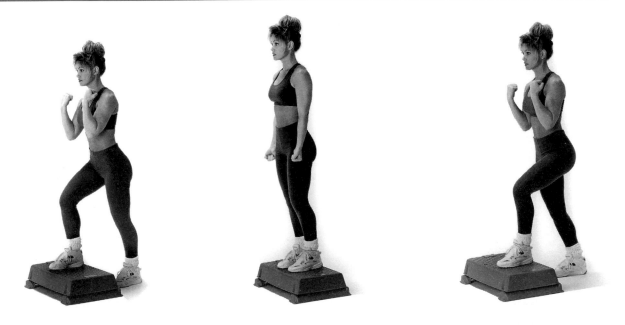

WORKOUT THREE: ADVANCED DAYS 1, 3 & 5

13. ALTERNATING KNEE LIFT *(p. 56)* **WITH OVERHEAD PRESS** *(p. 86)*

1 repetition

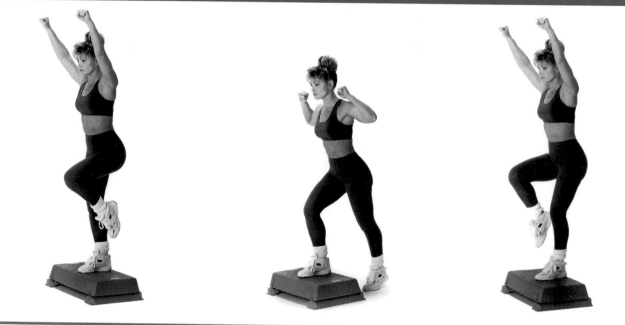

14. BASIC LEFT *(p. 46)* **WITH ALTERNATING BICEPS CURL** *(p. 83)*

3 repetitions

Repeat exercises 12–14 in sequence 4 times.

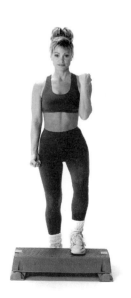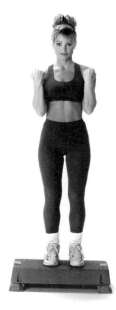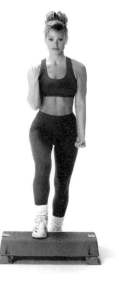

STEP PATTERNS

15. OVER THE TOP
(p. 64) **WITH OVER-**
HEAD PRESS *(p. 86)*
3 repetitions

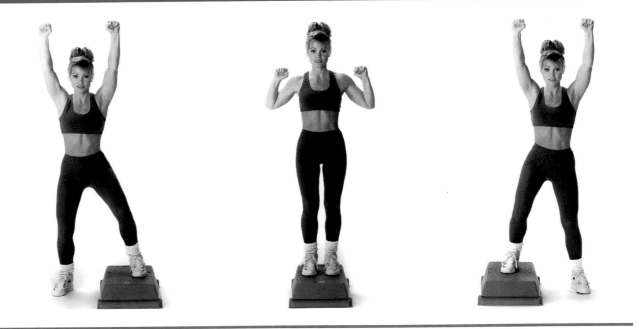

16. TURN *(p. 62)*
WITH CHEST CROSS-
OVER *(p. 92)*
3 repetitions

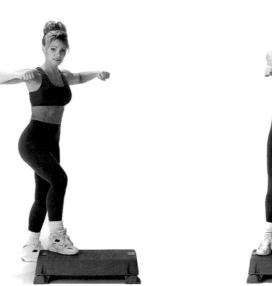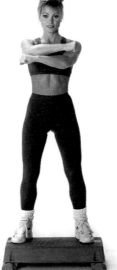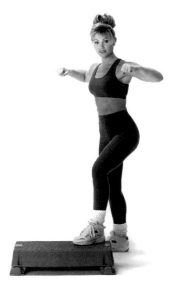

WORKOUT THREE: ADVANCED DAYS 1, 3 & 5

17. OVER THE TOP
(p. 64) **WITH**
OVERHEAD PRESS
(p. 86)
3 repetitions

Repeat exercises 15–17
in sequence 4 times.

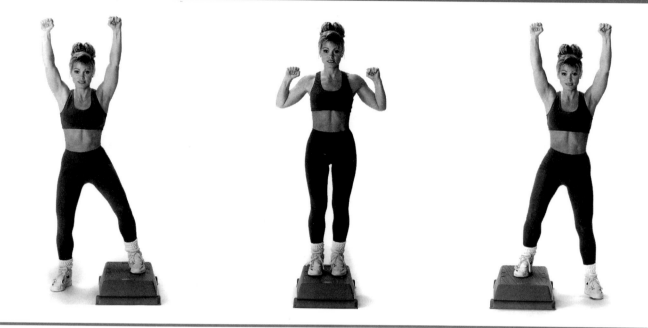

18. TURN *(p. 62)*
WITH CHEST
CROSSOVER *(p. 92)*
3 repetitions

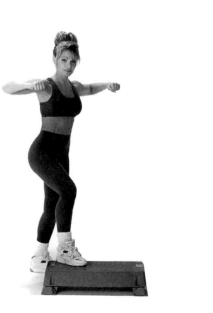
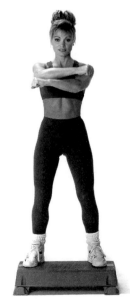
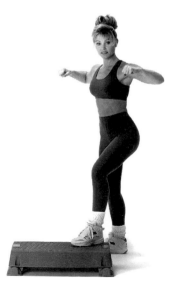

STEP PATTERNS

19. ACROSS THE TOP *(p. 76)* **WITH OVERHEAD PRESS** *(p. 86)* 3 repetitions

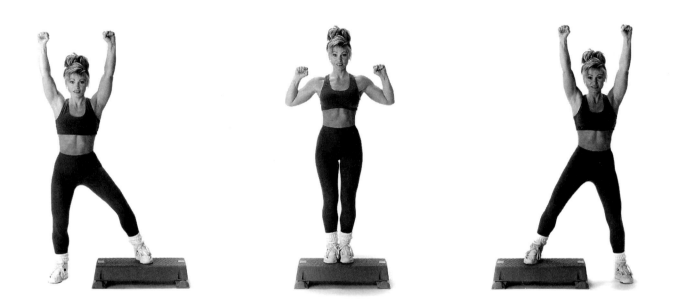

20. ALTERNATING KNEE LIFT *(p. 56)* **WITH SHOULDER PUNCH** *(p. 85)* 1 repetition

Repeat exercises 18–20 in sequence, 4 repetitions

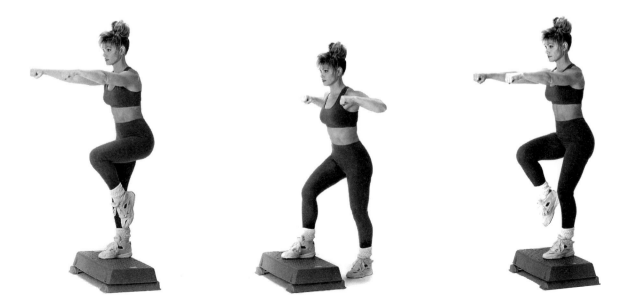

WORKOUT THREE: ADVANCED DAYS 1, 3 & 5

21. ALTERNATING BACK LUNGE *(p. 70)* **WITH CHEST CROSSOVER** *(p. 92)*
8 repetitions

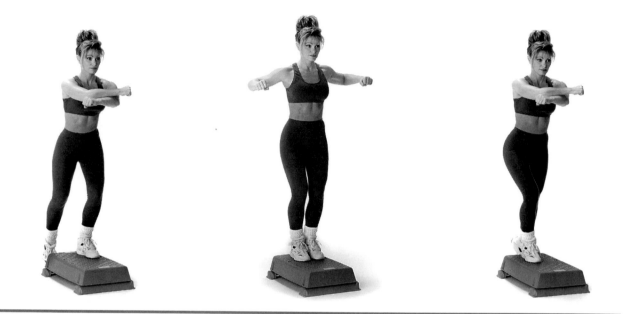

22. STRADDLE DOWN *(p. 72)* **WITH TRICEPS KICK BACK**
(p. 90) 4 repetitions

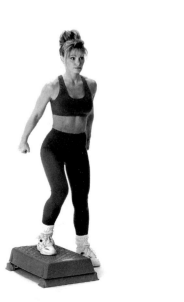 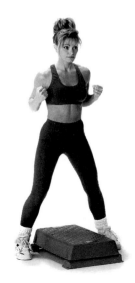 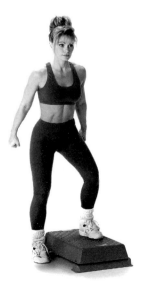

STEP PATTERNS

23. ALTERNATING LUNGE *(p. 70)* WITH CHEST CROSSOVER
(p. 92) 4 repetitions

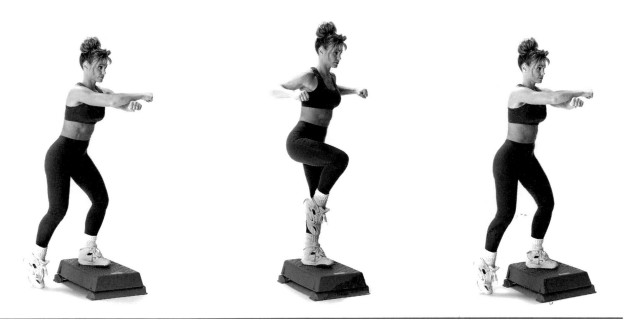

24. BASIC RIGHT *(p. 44)* WITH BICEPS CURL *(p. 82)*
3 repetitions

Repeat exercises 21–24 in sequence 4 times.

Repeat exercises 1–24 in sequence.

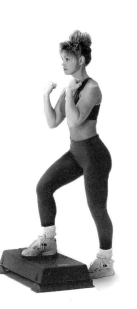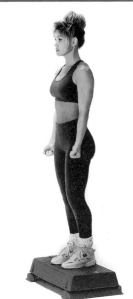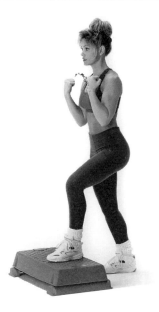

WORKOUT THREE: ADVANCED DAYS 2, 4

DAYS 2, 4 BODY-SCULPTING SEQUENCE

OUTER LEG LIFT
(p. 101)

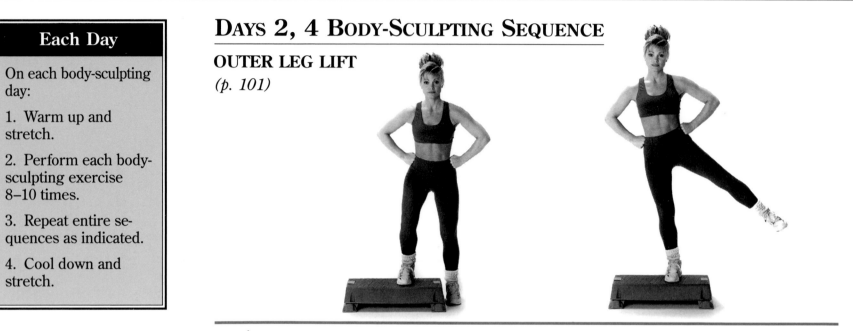

PLIÉ *(p. 99)*

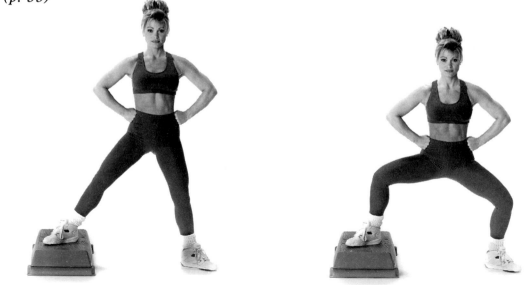

BODY-SCULPTING EXERCISES

SINGLE-LEG SQUAT
(p. 100)

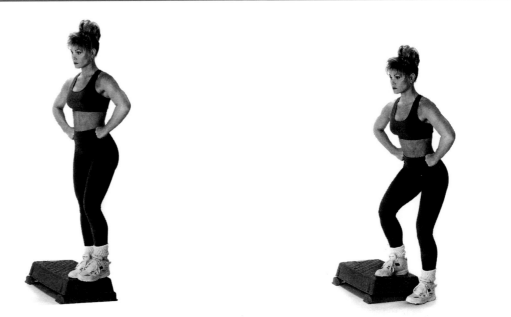

ALTERNATING LUNGE *(p. 98)*

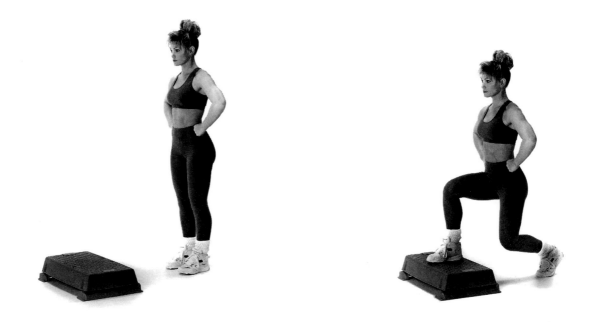

WORKOUT THREE: ADVANCED DAYS 2, 4

HAMSTRING HEEL
PRESS *(p. 102)*

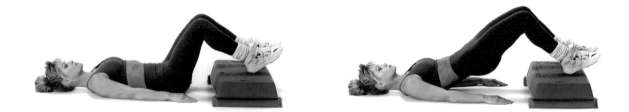

PUSH-UP *(p. 103)*

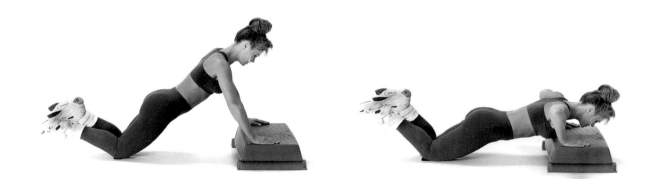

BODY-SCULPTING EXERCISES

TRICEPS PUSH-UP
(p. 104)

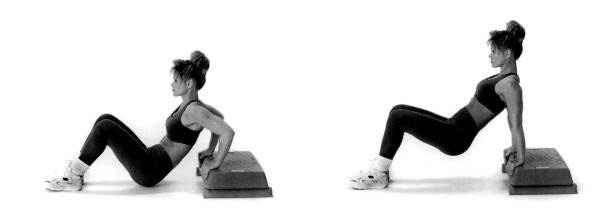

REVERSE ARM LIFT
(p. 105)

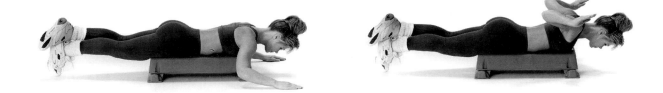

WORKOUT THREE: ADVANCED DAYS 2, 4

**ABDOMINAL
CROSSOVER** *(p. 107)*

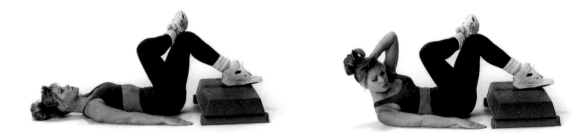

OVERHEAD PRESS
(p. 109)

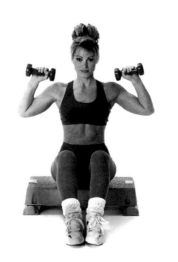 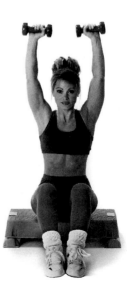

BODY-SCULPTING EXERCISES

BICEPS CURL
(p. 108)

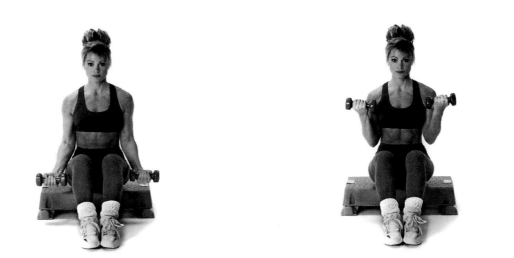

ABDOMINAL LIFT
(p. 106)

Repeat exercises in
sequence 3 times.

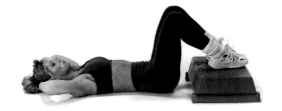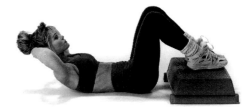

EPILOGUE: EXERCISE RISKS

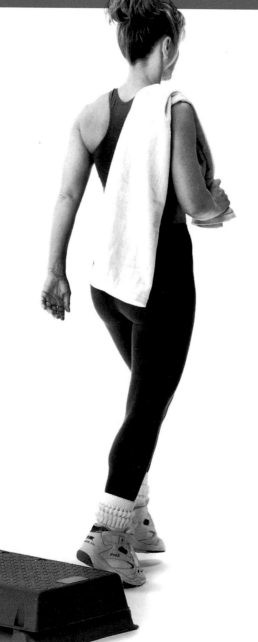

The days of "no pain, no gain" are gone. It is acknowledged that if exercise makes you hurt, something is wrong.

If you're aware of your body and its limits and you pay attention as you exercise, you can pace your workout with your level of conditioning. Much of the risk of injury can be avoided. However, you must keep in mind that accidents, like a slip and fall or a twisted ankle, can happen if you're not careful.

So if you are generally healthy and have no reason to suspect otherwise, a controlled exercise program is not likely to be a health risk. But if you know or suspect that you have any condition that might be aggravated by exercise, you should be cautious. If there's any question in your mind about your ability to exercise aggressively, get a medical check-up before you begin.

Be aware of your body and it's limits so that you can enjoy all the benefits of exercise.

Danger Signs

If you experience any of the following symptoms after you begin exercising, stop at once and see your physician before resuming.

- Chest pains
- Severe discomfort anywhere
- Illness or nausea
- Difficulty in breathing
- Dizziness or disorientation
- Numbness in any part of your body

In addition, observe these precautions when exercising:

- Reduce or avoid exercise in extreme heat or cold.
- Reduce or stop your activity if you start feeling uncomfortably tired while exercising.
- Don't suddenly increase your exercise rate, duration, or complexity; make all such changes gradually as you become conditioned to handle the increase.
- Don't exercise if you're not well.

Look for Tamilee's videos wherever videos are sold,

or call 1-800-453-6868.

Want to spend more time working out with Tamilee Webb? Check out her new video fitness series, *Building Tighter Assets,*™ and her first at-home exercise book, *Tamilee Webb's Original Rubber Band Workout.*

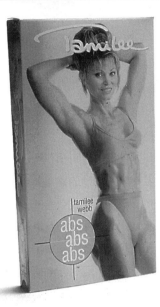

Abs, Abs, Abs™

Three 15-minute programs for a great workout.
($14.95)

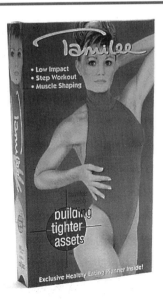

Building Tighter Assets™

Head-to-toe fat burning and muscle toning.
($19.95)